$\mathcal{R}$ENDEZ**VOUS**
Exciting Him

The Steps Women Want for Creating The Habits Needed for Living The Romantic Lifestyle ...More Joy, Harmony, Fun, Non-Sexual & Sexual Romance, and Success in Your Committed Relationship

BENILDA NYA GUERRERO-ORTEGA

authorHOUSE®

AuthorHouse™
1663 Liberty Drive
Bloomington, IN 47403
www.authorhouse.com
Phone: 1-800-839-8640

Published by AuthorHouse 12/18/2012

ISBN: 978-1-4567-6479-1 (sc)
ISBN: 978-1-4567-6478-4 (hc)
ISBN: 978-1-4567-6477-7 (e)

How to Order

www.rendezvousexcitinghim.com and rendezvouspleasingher.com

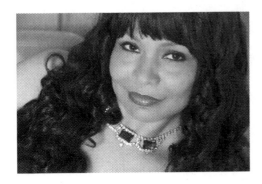

Dedication

To all the couples that are in love and have made a commitment to one another.

I also dedicate this book to Carlos Ortega; my awesome husband, my partner in life, my confidant and constant encourager. Together, we have braved many storms and our faith, love and mutual respect for each other always helps us persevere. Forever Yours!

Table of Contents

Introduction

With today's wealth of knowledge available on relationship skills, I am delighted that you have chosen to invest in this rendezvous reference book. You have made a winning decision!

I've written this book in honor of marriage, committed relationships and life, and it is written in two convenient versions: "His" and "Hers." These books are chock-full of encouragement, helpful ideas, inspiration and support that interact with each other. I recommend that each of the spouses (your partner in life) have their own version so that you can be assisted and coached simultaneously.

With each Weekly and Daily Coaching you'll find awesome assistance for a happier relationship with your mate and children as well as for your personal and professional life.

I am not suggesting that you become someone that you are not; I'm simply inviting you to stir up your romantic side and develop a new outlook so that you may enjoy the "Forever Pleasure and Excitement" that happen when you give romance the importance that it should have.

How to Use This Book

Take a moment to get acquainted with all that's here so that you can be aware of what's right at your fingertips when you need it. This book will become your journal and rendezvous reference book. It is the type of book that you'll want to carry with you everyday, like your appointment book.

In Part One of this book you'll find knowledge for understanding romance and its basics. There is a place to write his favorite things as well as ideas for romantic quickies, wedding anniversary gifts, ways to celebrate him every month, creative gifts and a suggestion for a very "exciting" night.

Part Two is where the majority of the coaching takes place. It is essential for both of you to be on the same week at the same time so that you can carry out the daily coaching practices together.

In Part Three you will be able to continue having fun on a monthly basis as you enjoy yourselves with different ways to take pleasure in monthly holidays and event coaching.

Part Four will assist you in giving and receiving the beautiful gift of Roses and other Flowers with more meaning and gratitude.

Part Five is very important because, you will be able to write more of your mate's favorite things. There will be no more guessing. You will get it right every time and this will show him that you do pay attention, even to the smallest of things.

In Part Six you have space to write all those important dates and contacts, as well as a place to write important notes.

In Part Seven I conclude my coaching by giving you more fuel to fan the flames of Romance with ideas for giving each other pet names, sweet or sexy expressions and how to say "I love you" in other languages as well as the all necessary "Pleasure/Excitement Vouchers."

Throughout this book I have provided space for you to put pictures of your spouse, yourselves and family. I hope this book becomes the essential "Romance Rendezvous Reference" that I intended for it to be – so that you can "forever" please and excite each other and live a happy and victorious life together.

Acknowledgments

I would like to thank the many men and women who took part in my romance research while I was working on this book.

I also want to thank Mary, Max, Celia and Joey whose big heart and dedication helped me in the final organization of the book format.

Additionally, I would like to thank ©Adrian Wilcox Photography for his generosity and great work on my author pictures. Also, Carlos Ortega and Julio Cesar for the photography that was done for this book, as well as the model Einar Soto and Marquita Whittingham for her editing talents.

Finally, I want to thank Virgie Broussard-Pradia, my dance teacher and mentor of many years whose creative writing and excellent talents have inspired hundreds of people. I adore her love for people and passion for life.

$\mathscr{P}$ersonal Data

NAME:_____

ADDRESS:_____

CITY & STATE:_____ZIPCODE:_____

HOME PHONE:_____CELL:_____

E-MAIL:_____

BIRTHDAYS – Spouse:_____Children:_____

WEDDING ANNIVERSARY:_____

FIRST DATE ANNIVERSARY:_____

IN CASE OF EMERGENCY CALL:

NAME:_____Phone:_____

ALLERGIES:_____

MEDICAL ALERTS:_____

BLOOD TYPE:_____

DOCTOR:_____Phone:_____

OTHER SPECIAL EVENTS:

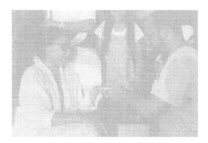

(Place an engagement or wedding picture of the two of you here.)

Part One

Understanding Romance
and
Romance Basics

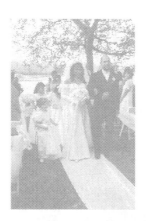

(Place one of your favorite wedding pictures here.)

"Romance"

The word "Romance," awakens different feelings and views in men and women.

Romance… The majority of women, no matter how beautiful and educated, yearn for a man that can understand her need for him to treat her with love, respect and kindness. A man that can help her feel unique and cared for. Someone who can give physical and mental interaction that does not always have to lead to sex.

Romance… For the majority of men, romance means physical and mental interaction that leads to sex, or a fairy-tale world that lives in movies and in novels. Some men and women think that it is something that it's not real or possible, and expensive to achieve.

Most women want and enjoy Non-sexual Romance anywhere and everywhere, but they must have their Sexual Romance as good as it can be… passionate foreplay and tender after-play.

Most men want and enjoy Non-sexual Romance anywhere and everywhere, but they must have their Sexual Romance as good as it can be… hot quickies and passionate lovemaking.

*K*nowing your mate's emotional state and religious beliefs will help you to appropriately give some thought to how your mate might react to these suggestions before trying them. Your spouse's state of mind and personality will help you to determine whether the attempt is appropriate for your marriage, or even worth the effort. Whatever you do, be sensitive!

*N*o matter how old you are or how long you've been together, you should create new ways and ideas to surprise your mate.

Benilda Nya

Essentials for Romance

Timing... You want to make sure that your spouse is available for the time you'll need for your display of non-sexual romance or passion for sexual romance. Communication with him will let you know if he has to work late or if he made other plans. It will also help you understand his needs: Would he rather stay home and eat a good home cooked meal or take out followed by a foot or full body massage before going to sleep, or to go out to eat followed by dancing – or would he prefer to have time alone? Will he enjoy a hot quickie or is he ready for passionate lovemaking?

Setting... The romantic atmosphere must consist of a variety of backdrops: lighting, mood, pleasant aroma, a clean and organized home, favorable conditions, as well as some inspiring music. Playing the romantic music that the two of you enjoyed when you were first attracted to each other and started dating, does wonders for renewing that exciting first time feeling. The "Setting," also includes an attractive you: having a fresh, clean and well groomed body, hands, feet and hair. When at home, wear nice or sexy loungewear, and dress very feminine or sexy when you go out with him. Dab on yourself the fragrance that he loves on you (lightly).

**To produce the best intensity for romance,
the setting must have...**

Passion... The passion for "desiring" and "yearning" someone is a strong force (you were introduced to these feelings when you first fell in love). That passion can create interest and diligence in you to master your touch, foreplay and sexual skills, making it incredibly electrifying for his body and soul.

Infuse passion with...

Pleasure... There is a pleasure that goes beyond loving one another. Delighting in each other is vital, taking satisfaction in the mastering of your non-sexual and sexual skills (this is not easy, and it requires daily nourishment). Make a decision to work as hard on your marriage as you do when you put in a 50/60 hour week at work. If you have accomplished great things in your professional life, make sure that you also are proficient in your private life. Take pleasure and pride in creating excellence in your marriage, as well.

Benilda Nya

Be His Romantic Heroine

Take time to explore and to fulfill the Sexual and Non-sexual Romantic desires in the man you love. The romantic heroine is a great lover because she doesn't just want pleasure for herself, but she also enjoys giving… visual, mental & physical pleasure to her man.

You can create this mood by…

- Getting rid of all the interruptions ahead of time.

- Stimulating his five senses: soft lighting, comfortable room temperature, soft/silky fabrics, touching him in the places that drive him wild, playing sexy music, using sensual aromas, putting on something to please his eyes.

- Looking at him with passion and desire: Smile with your eyes, make eye contact and keep looking at him when he is talking to you.

- Great kissing: Sensual soft kisses and HOT, Passionate ones, as well.

- Using sweet talk/sexy talk: speak with a soft, low voice; use passionate words that let him know how much you want him. Keep the spotlight on him, what you love about his body, how good it feels, the way it smells, and the way it responds to your touch and kisses. Tell him how you want to make love to him.

- Use words that let him see and feel that you are enjoying every moment with him. Don't talk about past or future things; keep your focus in the present, enjoying the moment. Other sweet talk topics consist of: nature, art, colors, literature, textiles, fashion, food and wine.

Benilda Nya

Make Way for the Good Habits that Support Romance

Non-sexual Romance is caressing and touching without expectations of a sexual interaction. This is kind of a confirmation of our capability of being concerned about the one we love.

Romantic Love is that unbelievable emotion of passion for someone. If you want that feeling to last a lifetime, you need to prevent hurting each other and try to fulfill each other's emotional desires as much as possible. Let's avoid being bankrupted in these areas by successfully making a daily deposit into this account.

The way a woman treats and understands her husband is very important in order for him to feel comfortable in communicating and connecting with her.

A man wants his wife to respect him, to enjoy loving him and giving him physical pleasure. You've got to make it good for him.

Benilda Nya

Distrust, Will Buy you a One-way Ticket to the Demise of Romance

Do not be a woman who is always calling her husband, getting upset if he does not check in every hour, or getting upset if he gives another woman a compliment. That kind of behavior will destroy your communication and connection and ultimately, his desire for being with you.

If he has done something or continually does things to deserve your distrust then the both of you need to work that out; if necessary, get some counseling. If in the past he did something that he has repented for and has asked you to forgive him, and if he has not violated your trust since, you really should let go of the past so that your future with him can be a peaceful and rewarding one.

Now, if you have been the one to abuse his trust, then you must repent and ask him to forgive you (if you have not already done so). If he is the one checking up on you all the time and you have already mended your ways, then you need to have a very serious conversation concerning his trust for you. You need to ask him; "What do you need for me to do to have you trust me?"

There is nothing worse than to live with someone that you can't or don't trust. Without trust it is impossible to have a relationship that is successful and pleasurable. So please, do not abuse and destroy the trust that your husband has in you. To get him to trust in you, you must be consistently honest on a daily basis in every area of your life. Even in the smallest of things, let integrity and excellence be your driving force.

To attract him more, you have to be trustworthy. You should also be able to understand and make provision for his physical, emotional, social, intellectual and spiritual needs. Be kind, patient and supportive and have a loving and positive attitude. Let him know how much you love, respect and value him by treating him like the king that he is.

Benilda Nya

Difficult To Romance?

Many married couples have a difficult time being romantic because they do not know how to enjoy each other. Even if they love one another, they just don't seem to have the desire or drive to please and honor each other. Other couple's passion begins to fizzle because of hurt, disappointment or monotony. Either way, they gradually fall apart due to years of, unfulfilled dreams and goals, bitterness or blame.

Other couples become nothing more than business partners who have to maintain their insignificant names ("Mr. and Mrs."), because they do not believe in divorce, or have to stay married because of family, professional, religious or social obligations; counseling maybe of some assistance for these situations.

Some spouses have a physical, mental or medical condition that prevents them from having a fulfilling sexual life with their mate. Please be patient, remember your vows/commitment to this wonderful person, and work on everything possible to find healing and restoration or work together to re-invent your sexual romance.

If you and/or your husband were virgins when you got married, I congratulate you. One of the best things about sexual purity is that you won't be comparing yourselves to anyone else. If you were not virgins, but decided to honor each other by waiting for sexual intimacy until your wedding night, I also congratulate you. It is not easy to have your favorite dessert in front of you and not taste or eat it. Whichever one is your situation, you will have your trials. Please, be patient with him and with yourself as you learn about each other.

In many of these cases my books: "RENDEZVOUS - Exciting Him," and "RENDEZVOUS - Pleasing Her," can be a great source of motivation and inspiration to help you and your spouse improve the quality of your marriage. With a positive mental attitude and the desire to improve the quality of your marriage, you can safely navigate to your destination... *Enjoying Each Other and Life Together.*

Benilda Nya

How well do you know him?

*B*y paying attention to him when he speaks and by watching his reactions to things, you will get most of the answers. The rest you will have to get by investigating or by asking him straight out, but please be careful not to give away too much so that you can still keep the element of surprise.

Favorite colors:_____

Type of music he likes:_____

Favorite mood lighting:_____

Favorite travel destinations:_____

Favorite hobbies:_____

Favorite retreat spots/hotels:_____

Surprise ideas:_____

Favorite gift ideas:_____

Favorite precious metals:_____

Favorite plants/herbs/flowers:_____

Favorite precious stones:_____

Favorite cologne:_____

Favorite candle/incense/aromatherapy:_____

Favorite sport(s) & teams:_____

What he likes least about himself/body:_____

_____

Lovemaking positions, places to make love:_____

_____

_____

What can you wear to turn him on:_____

_____

What does he consider romantic?_____

_____

_____

Favorite place to shop:_____

Clothing & shoe styles/designers:_____

Clothing/shoe size:_____

Favorite accessories:_____

Favorite spa/salon/barber:_____

Favorite toothpaste/soap/shampoo:_____

_____

Favorite books/authors:_____

_____

Best friends:_____

Favorite movies/TV shows:_____

_____

Favorite animals/cartoon:_____

Dream car:_____

Dream house (where, what kind, what would it look like):_____

_____

Favorite Style of Furniture/home accessories:_____

_____

Pet peeves:_____

Things that are embarrassing to him:_____

_____

Favorite TV personality likes/dislike:_____

_____

Favorite influential people:_____

Favorite perfume he loves on you:_____

Clothing styles he likes to see you in (for: play, casual, dressy, business):

_____

Things he likes/dislikes about you:_____

_____

Favorite Holiday/time of year:_____

His work schedule:_____

Where he parks at work:_____

Favorite restaurants:_____

_____

Favorite foods:_____

_____

Favorite desserts:_____

Favorite fruits/nuts:_____

Favorite candies/chocolates:_____

Favorite beverage/wine/champagne:_____

His worst fear(s):_____

Things he dislikes:_____

Favorite way to relax/de-stress:_____

_____

Other special interests:_____

_____

_____

_____

See page 195 - Part Five: for more of his "Favorite Things" to fill in.

Benilda Nya

Romantic Quickies
(Non-sexual)

- Always walk in to a party, restaurant or special event arm in arm.
- **Give him a call during the day just to tell him that you miss him and you can't wait for him to get home.**
- Tell him "I love you." Or "I'm so in love with you."
- **Make the morning coffee, tea or juice and bring it to him served on your fine china.**
- Set the table beautifully for breakfast, lunch or dinner.
- **Wake him up with kisses.**
- Ask him in the morning what he would like to have for dinner.
- **Flirt! Blow him a kiss from across the room. Wink at him. Pinch him.**
- Get his clothes ready for work (be his personal fashion stylist).
- **When you do the laundry, press his pants, starch and press his shirts.**
- At night when you are going to sleep, cover him, kiss him goodnight and massage his feet.
- **On a cold winter night, make some hot cocoa or tea for both of you, cover yourselves with a blanket, cuddle on the couch and watch TV.**
- On a hot summer day/night, make some lemonade or iced tea and serve it to him.
- **Thank and praise him for his chivalry.**
- Once in a while, sit down with him to watch his favorite sports team play. Serve some snacks, beverages and root along with him.
- **Surprise him with tickets to go see his favorite sports or hobby event.**
- Is he working hard to achieve a goal? Has he accomplished a goal or dream? Tell him that you are proud of him.
- **Keep a clean home.**
- Decorate your home (especially the bedroom and bathroom) with a romantic touch.
- **When you are home, relax and wear pretty "Loungewear."**

Benilda Nya

Romantic Quickies

(Sexual)

WARNING: some may consider some of these suggestions offensive.
Knowing your mate's emotional state and religious believes will help you to *appropriately* give some thought to how your mate might react to these suggestions before trying them. Your spouse's state of mind and personality will help you to determine whether the attempt is appropriate for him, please be sensitive!

- ❤ **Give him a call during the day and tell him what you are going to do to him tonight or what you want him to do to you.**
- ❤ Tell him, "Come here; I want to give you some lip service," then kiss him passionately all over his body.
- ❤ **Make the morning coffee, tea or juice and bring it to him served on your fine china, in your birthday suit. (Please use caution while carrying anything hot.) Then give him a morning quickie.**
- ❤ When you sit down to eat at the dinner table (at home and alone with him), wear a top that shows your cleavage (really low and daring).
- ❤ **Wake him up by whispering sexy things in his ear.**
- ❤ Dance for him: sensual belly dance, a chair dance or dance sexy to the music that turns him on.
- ❤ **Meet him for "lunch," at the nearest hotel from his job. Prepare his favorite foods and bring it in a picnic basket.**
- ❤ Make love to him in the middle of the afternoon.
- ❤ **If you own a swimming pool and have privacy in it: On a hot summer night, invite him for a skinny dip. If you do not have a swimming pool, then fill up your bathtub and take a long sensual bath together.**
- ❤ Go to a drive in movie, and while watching the movie take delight in touching and kissing each other.
- ❤ **Serve dinner in high heels and just the apron, or wear sexy lingerie or "easy access" loungewear.**

(As always, please make sure that you have privacy when you want to enjoy some indoor/outdoor sexual romance.)

Benilda Nya

Wedding Anniversary Gifts

	TRADITIONAL	MODERN
FIRST	Paper	Clocks
SECOND	Cotton	China
THIRD	Leather	Crystal/Glass
FOURTH	Fruit/Flowers	Appliances
FIFTH	Wood	Silverware
SIXTH	Candy/Iron	Wood
SEVENTH	Wool/Copper	Desk Sets
EIGHTH	Bronze/Pottery	Linens/Lace
NINTH	Pottery/ Ceramic	Leather
TENTH	Tin/Aluminum	Diamond Jewelry
ELEVENTH	Steel	Fashion Jewelry
TWELFTH	Silk/Linen	Pearls
THIRTEENTH	Lace	Textiles/Fur
FOURTEENTH	Ivory	Gold Jewelry
FIFTEEN	Crystal	Watches
TWENTIETH	China	Platinum
TWENTY-FIFTH	Silver	Silver
THIRTIETH	Pearl	Diamond
THIRTY-FIFTH	Coral	Jade
FORTIETH	Ruby	Ruby
FORTY-FIFTH	Sapphire	Sapphire
FIFTIETH	Gold	Gold
FIFTY-FIFTH	Emerald	Emerald
SIXTIETH	Diamond	Diamond

Please do not forget to give him a card; whether you buy it or whether you make it, the card should never be skipped.

Happy Anniversary Sweetheart

For your Wedding Anniversary you can be as creative as possible; whether you have fifty dollars, five hundred, five thousand dollars or more (save money for especial occasions), the idea is to make it special, thoughtful and romantically memorable.

Example

For your first wedding anniversary, you can give him a beautiful clock with an inscription like: "Thank you, baby, for a beautiful time in this first year of our marriage." Your wife who adores you, _____.

Or...

You can go and get some sexy pictures taken. Use a female photographer that agrees to use your own camera so that you can keep and have all the rights to your pictures. You could also have one of your creative female friends take the pictures with your camera. You can copy some poses from some of the pictures/calendars of popular sex symbols of the past or present, wear some similar clothing, get your hair and make up done right (very sexy). Then take a couple of the sexiest pictures and make them into wallet size, write on the back something like; "One HOT year," "One HOT wife." Love _____, and laminate them. Buy him a large wedding anniversary card and put the pictures inside of it, write on the card; "look at them during the day and think of me."

You can also make those same pictures into large size posters (20X18) autograph them and display them on a couple of art easels with balloons hanging from the top of them in the living room, so that he sees them the second he walks in the house. Wear one of the outfits in the pictures (hair and make up too) with your high heels and greet him with "Happy Anniversary Darling." After dinner you can give him the card with the wallet size ones.

(If he is taking you out, after the sexy surprise, you are ready to get into your dress and go when he is ready.)

*W*hat ever you decide to do for the anniversary, do it with thoughtfulness and with serious memories and romance in mind to fit your husband's character.

Benilda Nya

Be Creative in Your Gift Giving

Take time and effort with the way you wrap and present the gift: use coupons to be redeemed, search and find, follow the trail, hot/cold, solve a mystery, take him out for dinner and have the waiter bring him the gift on a dessert platter. There are also different reasons why you are giving him a gift, and there are many kinds of gifts that you can give to him, for example: A comical gift, Cultural, Spiritual, Homemade or Custom-made, Big or Small, Inexpensive/Expensive, Sexy/Conservative, Romantic/Practical or to congratulate him on a Social or Professional achievement. You have a lot to choose from, so it does not have to be expected or boring.

For his birthday, give him a gift or surprise him with something really extraordinary each day for the whole birthday month. If it is proper for both of you, give him a "Theme Party." Example: a "Hafla," which is an Arabic themed party with Middle Eastern music; live or with a DJ who specializes in Middle Eastern music, belly dancers taking turns performing and some open-floor dancing for everyone else. Your husband will feel like the king that he is.

Benilda Nya

Every month you have an opportunity to celebrate him with a gift. If he enjoys flowers, give him a masculine flower arrangement with the flower of the month or you could give him jewelry with the stone of the month and its meaning. Give him the flowers in different designs and sizes. For his birthday, you could also give him jewelry with his birthstone.

January
Flower: Carnation, Snowdrop
Birthstone: Garnet–constancy
-**Celebrating Tip**
On the second week of the month, send him a beautiful arrangement of carnations and snowdrops.

February - Make this, a Valentine's Month, not just Day
Flower: Violet, Primrose, Begonia
Birthstone: Amethyst–sincerity
-**Celebrating Tip**
Give him a pair of amethyst cuff links, and write him a little love note thanking him for his sincerity.

March
Flower: Daffodil, Jonquil
Birthstone: Aquamarine, Bloodstone–courage
-**Celebrating Tip**
On the second week of the month, give a small arrangement of the two flowers for his desk.

April
Flower: Sweet Pea, Daisy
Birthstone: Diamond–innocence
-**Celebrating Tip**
Give him a diamond pinky ring.

May
Flower: Lily of the Valley, Lily
Birthstone: Emerald–love, success
-**Celebrating Tip**
Send him a very masculine arrangement of Lilies.

June - National Rose Month
Flower: Rose
Birthstone: pearl, alexandrite, moonstone–health

Roses date far back to pre-historic days. They are more than 33 million years old and have been used among friends and lovers to send all sorts of messages, and they are used for many reasons.

-Celebrating Tips
1. On June 1st, send him 10 (yellow & orange) Roses. Let the card say: "Passionate thoughts of you… my perfect 10."

2. End Rose Month by preparing a luxurious and romantic bubble bath for the both of you. Let a poster size note greet him at the door with instructions to follow the rose petal trail (frame the poster with roses). Let the rose petal trail lead to the bathroom where you have candlelight, music, finger food and some champagne, sprinkle the bubble bath with lots of rose petals. Caress and kiss him, have a flirtatious conversation as you wash and feed each other. Make yummy and passionate love to him.

Famous Rose Quotes
- What's in a name? That which we call a rose/By any other name would smell as sweet. – William Shakespeare, Romeo and Juliet act II, sc. ii
- O, my love's like a red, red rose/That's newly sprung in June. – Robert Burns, A Red, Red Rose
- Rose is a rose is a rose is a rose. – Gertrude Stein, Sacred Emily (1913), a poem well used in Geography and plays.

See Part Four: Flower Meaning (pg 183), for the meaning of the color and story of roses, as well as other flower meanings.

July
Flower: Larkspur, Water Lily, Sunflower
Birthstone: Ruby – contentment
-Celebrating Tip
Give him a ruby necktie clip.

August
Flower: Gladiolus, Poppy
Birthstone: Jade, Peridot, Sardonyx – married, happiness
-Celebrating Tip
If this is his birthday month, celebrate him by giving him a jade, peridot or sardonyx bracelet with a beautiful card expressing how happy he makes you.

September
Flower: Aster, Pansy
Birthstone: Sapphire–clear thinking
-Celebrating Tip
On the second week, give him the flower of the month.

October
Flower: Magnolia
Birthstone: Opal, Tourmaline–hope
-Celebrating Tip
Give him an opal ring

November
Flower: Chrysanthemum, Orchid
Birthstone: Topaz–fidelity
-Celebrating Tip
Give him a desk size arrangement of chrysanthemums.

December
Flower: Hibiscus, Holly, Poinsettia
Birthstone: Turquoise, Zircon - prosperity
-Celebrating Tip
Give him turquoise cuff links as part of his Christmas gift.

See Part Three: Monthly Holidays and Events Coaching (pg 145) for more celebrating tips.

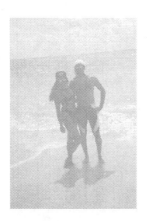

(Place a picture here from when you first met)

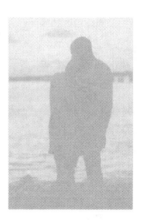

(Place a "Romantic" picture of the two of you here.)

Night of Passion (Suggestion for a very "exciting" night)

(WARNING – some of the language and suggestions contained in the night of passion suggestions, might be offensive to some.)

Knowing your mate's emotional state and religious believes will help you to *appropriately* give some thought to how your mate might react to these suggestions before trying them. Your spouse's state of mind and personality will help you to determine whether the attempt is appropriate for him, please be sensitive!

Greet him at the door (all dolled up: his favorite hair style, makeup, nail color, fragrance, wearing sexy loungewear) and kiss him on the lips. Then gently caress his face, lips and the back of his neck. Look into his eyes and tell him how "hot" and "handsome" he is; kiss him.

Start undressing him at the door, but leave on his pants; take him by the hand into the bathroom where you have prepared a candle lit bubble bath (just for him this time, not both of you), his favorite music, fruit/appetizer, and his favorite beverage. Then hand feed him a bite, while he chews continue to completely undress him. Ask him to step into the tub, while he steps in you go ahead and have a bite (of the fruit or appetizer), give him his beverage glass, you take yours and make a toast (To the most sexy, wonderful, amazing lover, etc.). After he takes a sip, feed him again and proceed to bathe him.

Continue to eat and drink as you bathe him. Be careful, you do not want this to end quickly. When done (after about 15-20 minutes) hand him a towel, and as he begins to dry himself off, go ahead and give him a kiss. Provide him with sexy loungewear for him to put on and take him to the dinner table (very beautifully set and with candlelight; do not forget to continue with the music). Serve one of his favorite dinners and dessert. During dinner, flirt with him and make sure that the conversation is romantic, passionate and sweet; feed him, touch him and look at him with bedroom eyes.

After dinner, take him to the "love nest," (a section in your living room, bedroom or by the fireplace that you have prepared with a furry throw rug, silky pillows and soft lighting). There you can serve dessert and persuade him to do a little slow dancing with you. While dancing, start undressing him, then sit him down and dance for him, finish it by making passionate love to him. (If you are not comfortable dancing for him, just slow dance with him and start touching and kissing him where and how he likes it as you remove his clothes and yours.)

During your lovemaking, tell him how good he feels. Take your time, and be very passionate. When he does something that pleases you, tell him how good it feels. If you want him to do something again, ask him. Express yourself!

After the point of ecstasy has been reached, spend time in after-play. Snuggle. Cuddle. Take hold of intimacy, and enjoy the present with him. Tell him how much he fulfills you, and that you love the way he takes care of you (and the kids if any). Fall asleep in each other's arms in your "love nest" (if possible)

In the morning, serve him breakfast in bed (or the love nest), have his favorite breakfast food and fruit. You can also have breakfast in bed with him. If things develop, make love to him again (in bed or in the shower).

Continue for the rest of the day with a positive and pleasant attitude. If it is a weekend day, go out and have some fun.

Do this according to his schedule. Make sure that he does not have to work late, that he's not concerned over a project deadline or that he has the time planned for something else. Call him at work (make it quick), and ask him for a date, then carryout your "Night of Passion" for that date.

If you have children you can plan for a baby sitter, friend or family member to take care of them for about 3-4 hours away from home or for an overnight stay. Make sure that the house is clean and tidy, smelling good, the "love nest" and dinner table are beautifully set, candles in place (please take caution with burning candles, make sure that they are in the proper containers and away from anything flammable, and that they will last for the time that you need them). Have the appetizer, dinner and dessert ready before he gets home. Time it just right so that the appetizer is not cold if it needs to be warm. You can keep the appetizer and dinner warm in a warming plate or oven (making sure that it does not dry out).

As he puts on his loungewear and combs his hair, you can rinse the tub a bit and blow out the bathroom candles. Clean up as you cook so that the dinner dishes are the only things left to clean, which you will do in the morning (tonight is about quality time). Remove your "love nest" before the kids get back.

Benilda Nya

Part Two

Pleasurable Weekly and Daily Coaching with Inspirational Sundays

For Monthly Holidays and Event Coaching,
Please See Part Three (page 145).

Select The Current Month, And Agree With Your Mate
To Do The Monthly Coaching Simultaneously.

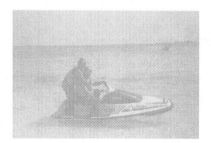

(Place a picture here of both of you doing something fun.)

$\mathcal{D}$ecide to fall in love all over again with your mate

....

$\mathcal{I}$t takes time to achieve greatness that can last a lifetime

....

$\mathcal{P}$ush yourself to greatness because you are lifetime partners

Benilda Nya

Sunday

A wife of noble (dignified, gracious, kind, good, courteous, gallant) character who can find? She is worth far more than diamonds and rubies. Her husband has full confidence in her and lacks nothing of value. Proverbs 31: 10-11

Monday

Say, "I love you" every hour that you are awake, but in a different language each time (see page 218 for saying I love you in other languages).

Tuesday

Stay in tune with your spouse's mood and needs to determine the appropriate romantic approach.

Wednesday

When he hugs you, thank him and tell him that in his arms you feel safe and secured.

Thursday

Get in the shower with him and surprise him with some quick pleasure.

Friday

When he kisses you, tell him how much you love his kisses.

Your physical movement will establish your mental outlook, so head up, shoulders back, stomach in.

Saturday

When he cooks or prepares something to drink, praise him. Do not complain about the mess he made or about the way he cleaned if it is not exactly how you like it done, and reward him when he does the laundry or cleans the house.

Use the pleasure vouchers in the back of this book.

NOTES/COMMENTS/JOURNAL: (Keep a record of what worked, changes made or new ideas.)

Daily Coaching – Week 1

*P*lay Together

On a stormy night, put a puzzle together or play…

Billiards

Dominos

Video Games

Board Games

*P*lay, *P*lay, *P*lay…

Golf

Tennis

Go Bowling

Hide–and Go Seek

Go to the park, ride a seesaw and swing together on the swings.

Benilda Nya

Prepared People Are Ready To Step Into Opportunity.

Sunday

Wise people store up knowledge... Proverbs 10: 14

Monday

Focus on what is good about your mate and marriage.

Tuesday

When he tells you sweet & beautiful things, tell him that you love the way he loves you.

Wednesday

Flirt with him.

Thursday

Call him at work and tell him that tonight you're going to let him give you all the loving.

Friday

Pursue him the way you did when you met him.

Saturday

Welcome and appreciate his spontaneity.

NOTES/COMMENTS/JOURNAL:

Daily Coaching – Week 2

Laughter is Healthy and Necessary in Every Relationship

*S*ome people are naturally playful; they know when to seize the moment to be amusing, while others have to decide to take a chance on the circumstances where humor can take place. A playful person can also make communicating very funny and exhilarating.

I encourage you to play and laugh together because it can be a very healthy factor in the development of a happy relationship. In a stressful moment it can help alleviate the situation and provide emotional relief. The rewards can be tremendous because it can help you to breakthrough the tough times of your relationship. So tickle him, act silly, tell him some good jokes or watch a funny movie together. If you have kids, include them in on the fun too.

Benilda Nya

If You Have To Debate Within Yourself To Do Right Or Not, You Do Not Have Any Principles.

Sunday

A man/woman who commits adultery lacks judgment; whoever does so destroys themselves and others. Pr. 6: 32 NIV

Monday

Touch him in a non-sexual way.

Tuesday

Never be a lazy lover; put some energy (more of yourself) into your lovemaking.

Wednesday

Tell him that you need him for a few minutes; when he's ready, hug and kiss him for a few minutes.

Thursday

Bag the nitpicking.

Friday

Tell him to sit back and enjoy the ride; you just want him to receive (a little bit of lovemaking).

Saturday

When he shares his intimate feelings with you, praise him and tell him that you love it when he tells you how he feels. Caress and kiss him afterwards.

NOTES:

Daily Coaching – Week 3

Do you want him to turn you on even more?

Encourage Him to be Sexy

Persuade him to wear nice or sexy loungewear around the house by buying some for him (visit my website: benildanya.com for store locations). If he speaks in a certain way that makes him sound sexy, tell him how you love it when he sounds like that!

Do you like to watch him undress? Tell him.

Does he have a great looking body or face? How about sexy eyes, lips or hands? Is he physically strong?

Praise him!

With your sincere praises, he can become sexier.

Benilda Nya

Nothing Significant Will Happen Until You Take The Initiative.

Sunday

…And the fool multiplies words. No one knows what is coming – who can tell him what will happen? Ecclesiastes 10: 14

Monday

Tell him that he is very handsome.

Tuesday

Treat his body like royalty.

Wednesday

Keep your word and promises to him and your children.

Thursday

Build him up. Show him that you are his #1 fan.

Friday

Tell him that you want to make love with the lights on (use soft lighting – rose or coral).

Saturday

Unconditionally accept each other.

NOTES/COMMENTS/JOURNAL: (Keep a record of what worked, changes made or new ideas.)

Daily Coaching – Week 4

De-stress Together

Boost immunity; live healthier, longer and happier

Meditate

....

Do Tai Chi

....

Practice Qigong

....

Stretch together

....

Go to your "Happy Place"

....

Get a manicure & pedicure

....

Do deep breathing exercises

....

Get restored & renewed with a massage

....

Take an aromatherapy bath with lavender oil

....

Do a 10-minute p.m. yoga de-stressor before going to bed

Benilda Nya

Teach Others How To Love You... Love Yourself.

Sunday

He who gets wisdom loves his own soul... Proverbs 19: 8

Monday

When he says sweet and loving things to you tell him: "You say all the words that my body and soul want to hear."

Tuesday

Return the touch... Touch him in a Non-sexual Romantic way every day, in different ways in public & private.

Wednesday

Go to sleep in each other's arms.

Thursday

Appreciate his compliments.

Friday

If he likes to watch you dress and undress, give him a show sometimes.

Saturday

Gaze into his eyes when you are out together.

NOTES:

Daily Coaching – Week 5

Greet him at the door with: "I want you NOW!"

This quick rendezvous can take place right in the foyer, living room, dining room or in the kitchen (make sure you have privacy).

This is a great way to show your appreciation for when he has done something that you love, whether it's giving you a gift or fixing something around the house, having a good attitude or showing physical expression. If you have children, get a baby sitter to take them for a walk or to the playground for the time you need. If you have other people living with you, then take it into your bedroom.

Benilda Nya

Love Him The Way He Wants And Needs To Be Loved.

Sunday

What a man/woman desires is unfailing love. Proverbs 19: 22

Monday

Let him delight himself in you. Do not rush him or deny him the pleasure.

Tuesday

Fondle him.

Wednesday

When he is romantic, thank him for it.

Thursday

Balance your lovemaking style. It shouldn't all be quickies, because you will discourage your mate. And neither should you have to exhaust yourselves in hours of sexual foreplay each time.

Friday

Make your own Romantic scene: kiss as you watch the sunset.

Saturday

Spend the day in bed; read, sleep, play cards/board games. Then take a shower or bath and go back to bed and have dinner in bed (order take-out and have it delivered).

NOTES/COMMENTS/JOURNAL: (Keep a record of what worked, changes made or new ideas.)

Daily Coaching – Week 6

Notice Him

A man loves it when the woman he loves becomes aware of his professional accolades, physical attributes and his efforts around the house, and she praises him about them. The incentive to train yourself to take notice is, that it will do wonders for the communication between the two of you, and it can also increase his help around the house.

Become aware of his Body

Appreciate his firm, fit, well-shaped areas and muscles. Does he have great looking hair or sexy baldhead? How about a firm/sexy/cute butt? Or does he keep his hands and nails clean and manicured? Are his feet free of bad odors? Is he free of the crotch itching habit that some men have? Is he neat? Does he dress well? Does he look good in a certain color or style? Praise and Compliment him. No matter what size he is, he can still be in great shape and look very handsome. Does he smell good? Compliment Him in a flirtatious way.

If he has gained a few pounds since you met him, do not criticize and put him down; instead help him to get back in shape. You both can start to exercise or get a personal trainer, and eat healthy (consult with your physician before starting any diet or exercise program).

Understand Him

A man loves it when the woman he loves becomes aware of the things that make him different from her, and she does not try to mold him into someone different or get offended by his differences. The incentive to train yourself in this area is that your relationship with him and the atmosphere of your home could be a more happy and peaceful one.

Benilda Nya

When You Love... You Are Happy To Give.

He who tends a fig tree will eat its fruit. Proverbs 27: 18

Enjoy kissing all body parts possible. You can do this in public (in non-sexual ways) and in private.

Enjoy him spoiling and babying you.

Touch him in a sexual way; tell him: "You are so hot."

Always appreciate and praise his way of surprising you.

Make out at the movies. Let him express his passion for you, and enjoy it.

Make "steamy" love to him in the shower.

Use the pleasure vouchers in the back of this book.

NOTES:

Daily Coaching – Week 7

Become aware of his Needs

Understand that his priorities are different than yours. Most men are hunters and problem solvers; they are trained to be efficient in the things of life; they are not trained to be housekeepers and to understand the female mind or hormonal changes. So be realistic and fair. Praise him for any and all efforts that he makes, especially when it comes to the house chores (yes, even if he does not do it the way that you do).

Verbalize it!

Do not get caught up in an attitude of nagging and complaining. That's the worst thing that can be done in a relationship. Information is communication, so when you want to have a heart to heart talk, tell him with a *pleasant* attitude that you need 30/45/60 minutes to talk to him (let him know when you would like this to take place; sometime today or before we go to bed, or ask, "when can we talk?"). Stick to the time you asked for.

If he does or says something that disappoints you or makes you angry, stop, count to ten, breathe slowly and deeply a few times before you act and speak. Ask him what he meant by what he said or did; ask him why he did not call to let you know that he was running late for dinner, etc. *Always* give him the chance to explain his actions before you allow your emotions to take action.

If you feel like there are not many good things to notice about him, think again. Could it be stress, the children, an unaccomplished goal/dream or maybe something in the marriage that has taken away your interest? What was it about him that attracted you when you first met him? If he has lost some of that spark, find out what you can do to help him get it back.

Benilda Nya

Sunday

Love is patient, love is kind. It does not envy, it does not boast, it is not proud. It is not rude, it is not self seeking, it is not easily angered, it keeps no record of wrongs. Love does not delight in evil but rejoices with the truth. It always protects, always trusts, always hopes, always perseveres. 1 Corinthians 13: 4-7

Monday

Exercise together.

Tuesday

Never say or feel that his compliments are not true. Believe him.

Wednesday

When he does something nice for you, tell him how good he is to you.

Thursday

Be consumed with his strengths.

Friday

Relax and debrief together from the stresses of the week: stretch and breathe in deeply.

Saturday

Feed each other while making love; sharing chocolate or chocolate covered fruits with champagne in a hot tub or in bed.

This is particularly great if you want to play a Greek night fantasy, or a Cleopatra and Anthony Egyptian night. With this beautiful world that God created with its vast selection of cultures, there are so many themes to choose from for sexual romance: Choose a different culture or Country every month to inspire your lovemaking.

NOTES/COMMENTS/JOURNAL: (Keep a record of what worked, changes made or new ideas.)

Daily Coaching – Week 8

❤ *G*ive him the confidence needed to look his best.

❤ *W*hen other attractive men are around; tell your husband/ your man: "you are so handsome/hot."

❤ *P*ersuade him to dress in the clothes that fit his fashion personality and body type.

Benilda Nya

How Do You Feel/Think About Yourself? ...You Are The Way You See Or Think About Yourself.

Sunday

As water reflects a face, so a man's/woman's heart reflects the man/woman. Proverbs 27: 19

Monday

Keep a clean, beautiful and inviting home.

Tuesday

If he looks good dressed up for work, tell him.

Wednesday

Play the music that helps both of you relax, and take an aromatherapy bath together.

Thursday

Realize the importance of good, sexual romance so that you can keep your husband craving for you.

Friday

Be thankful for the sweet things that he does for you.

Saturday

Break out the bubbly for dinner.

Keep a good stock of wine and champagne in your house (replace with alcohol free if you don't drink liquor).

NOTES:

Daily Coaching – Week 9

Getting to Know You

Are you...

Sad

Sick

Bored

Hungry

Worried

Fatigued

Overloaded

Overwhelmed

Do you have Low Self Esteem?

Arguments or discontent tend to increase rapidly when one of these physical and mental factors is present. Become aware of these issues and help him to understand your needs, so that he can be especially sensitive and comprehend your mood and if possible fulfill your desires. You can give him insight on how to lend a hand and assist you in a quick recovery.

Wisdom in the basic skills of communication, conversation and relationships will help you choose the emotional ambiance you would like in your relationship and in your home.

Benilda Nya

Be A Woman Of EXCELLENCE!

Sunday

Like a gold ring in a pig's snout is a beautiful woman who shows no discretion. Pr. 11: 22 NIV

Monday

Caress him.

Tuesday

Hug and kiss him, and tell him that you love him and to have a great day.

Wednesday

Empower yourself; learn to be a great lover. Learn what to do to his body by exploring it and asking him what he likes.

Thursday

After dinner, let him clean up the kitchen, then cuddle and talk and/or listen to music.

Friday

Ask him to meet you at his favorite four-or five-star hotel (your treat). Request an early check-in, bring a change of clothes for both of you and spend the night. ENJOY!

Saturday

Follow his lead.

NOTES/COMMENTS/JOURNAL: (Keep a record of what worked, changes made or new ideas.)

Daily Coaching – Week 10

Getting To Know Him

Is he...

Sad

Sick

Bored

Hungry

Worried

Fatigued

Overloaded

Overwhelmed

Does he have Low Self Esteem?

Arguments or discontent tend to increase rapidly when one of these physical and mental factors is present. Becoming aware of these issues will help you to be especially sensitive and understanding about what his need is, and in how you speak to him and what you can talk to him about. It will also give you insight on how to listen to him, and help you to understand his state of mind.

You can also help him by finding a way to alleviate the problem. You might need to give him time alone, or he might need some extra pampering or maybe even a pep talk.

Benilda Nya

SUCCESS Only Comes Before Work In The Dictionary.

Sunday

He who works his land will have abundant food. Proverbs 12: 11

Monday

Share his excitement in the things that excite him.

Tuesday

Meet him for lunch.

Wednesday

*Honor him by listening to what he has to say and understand him.
Express your feelings about something that is bothering you (in a
respectful, non-condemning way).*

Thursday

Tell him "I love you."

Friday

*Surprise him with 2 Or 3 tickets to his favorite sport team game (for him a
couple of friends).*

Saturday

*Do not over spend when he takes you shopping; stick to the budget that he
has set aside for you.*

NOTES:

Daily Coaching – Week 11

*G*o out on a date at least once a week. Have fun
the way you used to when you were dating.

(If you have children, plan for this according to their ages.)

Benilda Nya

Do What Is Right Even If No One Is Watching.

Sunday

A wife of noble character is her husband's crown, but a disgraceful wife is like decay in his bones. Pr. 12: 4 NIV

Monday

Play as hard as you work.

Tuesday

Become masterful in the bedroom. Excel in all areas of womanhood. Do not use sex to control your man; use sex to serve him and to give him and yourself pleasure. Do it well!

Wednesday

Kiss him, hug him, squeeze him and please him.

Thursday

Learn to belly dance.

Friday

Before he goes to bed, prepare a relaxing bubble bath for him. Serve him his favorite beverage.

Saturday

Be ready and willing for TLC.

NOTES/COMMENTS/JOURNAL: (Keep a record of what worked, changes made or new ideas.)

Daily Coaching – Week 12

$\mathcal{M}$arriage will challenge your ability to be resilient; it will dare your imagination to come up with positive resolutions. For a successful marriage, sometimes you will need to put your mate's satisfaction before your own. The denial of self is a great way to convey your love for your spouse.

$\mathcal{A}$s you nurture your relationship, be independently strong as you also depend on each other for certain things.

$\mathcal{T}$he bonds of holy matrimony sometimes entail pain and struggle, and the restraint and effort that are analogous to our pedagogical and professional development. But it is also rewarded with the satisfaction of achieving your goals and making your dreams a reality.

$\mathcal{S}$o go ahead and walk that extra mile and do those special things for your spouse, the reward of "absolute pleasure" is well worth it.

Benilda Nya

"Most Folks Are About As Happy As They Make Up Their Minds To Be."
– Abraham Lincoln

Sunday

For as he thinketh in his heart, so is he… Proverbs 23: 7

Monday

Round out your rough edges.

Tuesday

Thank and praise him for being thoughtful and romantic.

Wednesday

Coordinate his clothes for work. Pinch his backside and kiss him goodbye.

Thursday

When he showers you with flowers and/ or gifts, tell him how awesome he is.

Friday

Go see a movie with some friends.

Saturday

Be easy going.

NOTES:

Daily Coaching – Week 13

$\mathcal{A}$bsolute pleasure also comes through the recognition, love and encouragement of your spouse. Do not be possessive or consider yourself the most important part of the marriage relationship. Leave the past behind; do not let it determine your future. Initiate what you want out of your marriage. Learn to celebrate your spouse instead of just tolerating him. Show your husband that your love has no restrictions to its staying power and no end to its hope; your love for him will survive everything!

(For your safety and well-being; in relationships where there is abuse, addictions or mental problems: no restrictions to staying power and hope, need to be re-evaluated.)

Benilda Nya

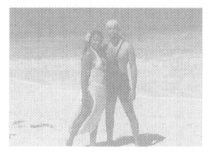

(Place a picture of the both of you here.)

Write down your goals and go over them daily. Take 2 - 3 minutes and see yourself accomplishing them and feel the way you will when they come to pass. This will increase your chances for achievement by more than 90%.

Sunday

Then the Lord replied: "Write down your vision, and make it plain on tables (paper), that he may run that readeth it. Habakkuk 2: 2

Monday

Romantic love is exclusive... Love, laugh, appreciate, understand and strive for excellence in everything you do for your mate.

Tuesday

Do not talk with him the way you talk with your girlfriends (as if he was a woman).

Wednesday

Cook for him his favorite breakfast. Kiss and hug him goodbye.

Thursday

When he hugs & kisses you, tell him that his love makes you rise above the stresses of the day. (His hugs and kisses should help you to feel that way.)

Friday

Use social and table etiquette in public. When he uses his social or table manners, tell him that his good manners make him extremely sexy.

Saturday

Take a motivational class together to increase your level of excitement in everything you do.
Use the pleasure vouchers in the back of this book.

NOTES/COMMENTS/JOURNAL: (Keep a record of what worked, changes made or new ideas.)

Daily Coaching – Week 14

While making love, tell him how much you want him.

Benilda Nya

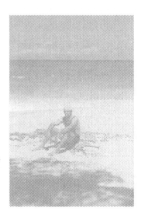

(Place a sexy picture of him here.)

Choices = Results... Please Do Not Make A Permanent Choice In A Short-Lived Situation.

Sunday

Like a bird that strays from its nest, is a man/woman who strays from his/her home. Proverbs 27: 8 NIV

Monday

Be a lady in public, but in the bedroom...you should be a seductress with your husband.

Tuesday

Be yourself. Talk to him about your feelings and ideas in a nice and non-confrontational manner.

Wednesday

Appreciate the way that he shows his love for you.

Thursday

Develop self-discipline, increase in knowledge regularly and expand your vocabulary.

Friday

Set the mood with candlelight, play music and dance for him.

Saturday

Get ready quickly for his spontaneity. Dress beautifully according to the event.

NOTES:

Daily Coaching – Week 15

What is it about him that turns you on?

Tell him.

Benilda Nya

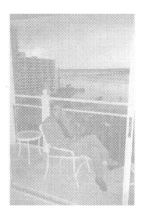

(Place another sexy picture of him here.)

Be RELENTLESS... When It Comes To Accomplishing Your Dreams, Goals, Purpose, Destiny And Your Happiness.

Sunday

A cheerful heart is good medicine, but a crushed spirit dries up the bones. Proverbs 17: 22

Monday

Believe in yourself. Focus on achieving your goals.

Tuesday

Give him "delicious" morning kisses.

Wednesday

Rekindle your desire and passion for your husband.

Thursday

Be open to his suggestions.

Friday

If he wants to take you out to a dance club or party, go.

Saturday

Make breakfast for the both of you, and eat breakfast in bed.

NOTES/COMMENTS/JOURNAL: (Keep a record of what worked, changes made or new ideas.)

Daily Coaching – Week 16

All About the Family

If you have children, you should develop a good relationship with them. You can play with them and depending on their age, teach them a game or sport. You could also take golf or tennis lessons together as a family. Maybe you can do a craft project or build something together.

Start this relationship when they're little so that you can have a better chance at those possibly trying teenage years.

The benefits are enormous because not only will you encourage and give your children the emotional and spiritual support that is essential for them to have, but you and your mate can also get pleasure from acting like kids again thus strengthening your romantic relations.

Teach your kids from an early age to be appreciative and thoughtful. Teach family values; encourage them to give gifts and cards to you, your husband, family and friends. They can design and make the cards and gifts or if they have a talent, encourage them to; write and sing a song, choreograph a dance, play their instrument, paint a picture or write a poem, etc.

Instruct and help your teenagers with their self-respect and help them with their self-esteem. Train your children to be self-sufficient and how to protect themselves and what to do in case of an emergency.

To understand each other's temperament better and to improve your communications, I recommend that you and your family take a test to find out the "personality type" of each of you.

Benilda Nya

Parents Are The Stage And Inspiration, For Their Children To Create On.

Sunday

Cook a nice Sunday dinner.

Train a child in the way he should go, and when he is old he will not turn from it. Proverbs 22: 6

Monday

Wakeup up grateful! Think of 3 things to be thankful for.
Before you go to sleep, think of at least 3 things that you are happy about and thank God for them.

Tuesday

Let him help with the kids.

Wednesday

Make a delicious breakfast, and eat together as a family.

Cook a delicious dinner and dessert; use your fine china and crystal.

Thursday

Meet him at the door when he comes home; kiss, and hug him, ask how his day was.

Friday

Let him do the laundry. Do not complain if he doesn't do it exactly like you.
Order his favorite takeout dinner. Praise him for taking care of the kids and/or the house.

Saturday

Arrange for privacy and after dinner, set the mood and belly dance for him.

NOTES:

Daily Coaching – Week 17

Is He A Dad?

Creating romantic moments takes on a whole new meaning when you have children. Your husband will still need TLC from you, and you will need a lot of patience. The children should be taught discipline and consideration from day one so that they can understand the need for Mom and Dad to have time alone. Do not hesitate to display non-sexual romance in front of your children. This will create a sense of security for the family: your boys will learn to be romantic, and the girls will appreciate and look for a man who will treat them well and is romantic. This will also help them in selecting a good mate and in having a successful relationship.

- ❤ The family should spend quality time together.

- ❤ The children will grow up and make a life for themselves, so make sure that you nurture your marriage with romance if you still want to have one after they leave.

- ❤ Give them (each of your children and your husband) your undivided attention, and tell them that you love them.

- ❤ You and your husband should agree on how to raise and discipline the children (never disagree on the method of discipline in front of the children).

Benilda Nya

Do Not Criticize Your Spouse Or Child Constantly. Instead Use The: "Positive" – "Negative" – "Positive" Method.

Sunday

He who heeds discipline shows the way to life, but whoever ignores correction leads others astray. Proverbs 10: 17

Monday

Group hug with the kids and husband; kiss them and tell them how much you LOVE them before they leave for work and school.

Tuesday

Always kiss him goodnight.

Wednesday

Call him during the day and tell him, "You are everything that a woman could hope for."

Thursday

It's a beautiful life. (You get what you say, what are you saying?)
Dress nice for dinner with Benilda Nya's "Loungewear Home-line," for women.

Friday

Cook his favorite dinner; buy his favorite dessert and beverage. Use your fine china and crystal, and light a few candles.
Show him your appreciation for all the wonderful things that he does to please you and to give you a good life.

Saturday

Enjoy being pampered.

Plan a homemade costume dinner party just for you guys. If you have children and they are old enough, get them involved too, and give away prizes for best costume, best creativity, color, etc (first, second, third, fourth, fifth place). Just make sure every body gets a prize. Let your child/ kids decide which award goes to Mom and Dad. Put your child/kids to bed, and then make it an "adults only" party in the bedroom. Leave on some soft lighting; make love to him with parts of your costume on. If you do not have children, after dinner dessert is "ON" you, make love to him on the dining room chair while you feed him "Dessert."

Daily Coaching – Week 18

If you are a mother, teach your children from a young age to be courteous and romantic.

♥ Teach your boy(s) how to give genuine compliments to their sister, aunties, grandmothers, and to their girl cousins. Instruct him/them on good manners, and social etiquette skills: to open doors and hold doors open for the ladies; to pull the dinner chair out if she is getting up, or push the chair in when she is sitting down, and to give a hand in carrying a shopping or grocery bag. Teach him/them to be neat and to help around the house. (He/they will also learn by watching your husband do these things.) Thank your child for being trustworthy and well behaved. Tell him "I love you," and how handsome he is.

♥ Praise your husband for being a good father. When he holds the door open, pulls or pushes in the chair for your daughter(s), when he brings or sends her favorite flowers or gives her a compliment, praise him for doing these things. Tell him how wonderful he is when he tells her that he loves her and that she is beautiful, smart or well behaved and thanks her for being trustworthy. Let him be attentive to her/their needs and wants. You should also tell your daughter these same things.

(Do this according to the age of your children.)

Benilda Nya

Discipline your son, and he will give you peace; he will bring delight to your soul. Pr. 29: 17 NIV

The righteous man leads a blameless life; blessed are his children after him. Pr. 20: 7 NIV

Your Attitude Makes A Big Difference.

Sunday

Everybody pitch in and cook a BIG breakfast: cook everybody's favorite food including those foods from your native Country (if other than American). Everyone also contributes in the clean up.
Better to live in a desert than with a quarrelsome and ill-tempered wife. Proverbs 21: 19

Monday

Go out for breakfast
Tell him that you LOVE him.

Tuesday

Let him get the kids ready for school.
Relax and enjoy the tenderness.

Wednesday

Let him do the laundry. Do not complain if he doesn't do it exactly like you

Thursday

If you need his help, ASK for it.

Friday

Before bed, light some candles, play romantic music and give him a sensual massage.

Saturday

Allow him to give you the day off, go and do what you want.

NOTES:

Daily Coaching – Week 19

If you are a mother, teach your children from a young age to be courteous and romantic.

❤ Enroll your children in etiquette classes; it will be one of the best investments that you can ever make for their future (please make sure that you also practice your manners with them and around them; be the example). Teach them to respect others and how to deal with difficult people. Do not spoil your children; you will just make it hard for them to succeed in life and function well in society.

❤ Remember that you and your mate are the ones that have the power to instill and create in your child/children the basic ingredients for a successful life. They are like a blank tape ready to record, therefore you greatly determine their values and character along with the social environment that you expose them to. Develop trust, learn to communicate well with your child/children and be an inspiration.

(Do this according to the age of your children.)

Benilda Nya

A good man/parent leaves an inheritance for his children's children. Proverbs 13: 22

Be very careful with the behavior that you accept from your child because, that is the behavior that you approve of.

Sunday

Folly is bound up in the heart of child, but *wise* discipline and correction will drive it far from him. Proverbs 22: 15

Monday

Kiss and hug and wish him a great day before leaving (if you have kids include them in also).

Tuesday

Take advantage of his erotic possibilities; touch, caress and kiss his skin.

Wednesday

Thank him for being thoughtful and tell him that you love him.

Thursday

Show him your appreciation… send him a singing telegram.
Let him check the kid's homework, and then, ask everybody (including your husband) to pickup a good book and read a couple of chapters (you should also join in and read your favorite book).

Friday

Take a walk hand in hand or go for a drive after dinner & tell him that he makes you feel special and beautiful. (Feel it & mean it.)

Saturday

Let him nurture you.

NOTES/COMMENTS/JOURNAL: (Keep a record of what worked, changes made or new ideas.)

Daily Coaching – Week 20

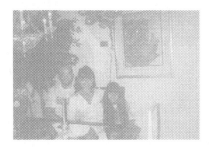

(Place your family picture here.)

Write Down Five Things That You Are Grateful For

1.

2.

3.

4.

5.

Think About These; Every Morning As Soon
As You Wakeup & Give Thanks.

To look the very best that you can look... Stay in Shape

*G*et a good night's sleep

....

Exercise three to five times a week

....

*E*at healthy and drink plenty of good water

....

For good health, stay within the desired weight for your height

....

*E*xercise your brain (learn a new hobby,
work on word or picture puzzles)

....

This regimen is great for anti-aging.

Take care of yourself; he needs you around for a long time, and he needs you to function well in spirit, body and soul.

(Consult with your doctor before beginning any form of diet and exercise.)

Benilda Nya

Connecting With Wise People Will Stimulate Your Imagination.

Sunday

He who walks with the wise grows wise, but a companion of fools suffers harm. Proverbs 13: 20

Monday

Give him a passionate kiss when he gets home, then; give him and yourself pleasure before bedtime!

Tuesday

Share your feelings openly instead of acting them out through whining or quarreling.

Wednesday

Call him during the day and talk sexy to him about what you want him to do to you / for you tonight.

Thursday

Devotion is essential for success. Devote yourself to your marriage.

Friday

Get dressed up for bed like you did for your honeymoon and stir up the flames of lust.

Saturday

Do not let him anticipate your moves; do something new to him, something totally unexpected.

NOTES:

Daily Coaching – Week 21

At the end of the day, both of you will need to recover from your day. Give yourselves thirty minutes to an hour to refresh and renew your spirit, body and soul. Talk it over with him to decide who goes first. Be kind. If you both need the same time off, then rotate and respect that time.

....

Start a book club. Take the family (spouse and children if old enough) to your favorite bookstore and find a book of your choice. Buy everybody his or her own book if you can. Designate a night during the week or weekend when everybody can take an hour or so to read their book (great family reading time). You can have your favorite dessert and beverages while you read (if you have only one book, you can rotate reading to each other).

Once a week over dinner you can discuss each chapter as it ends, until the book is finished. As you start a new book let another family member choose the next book. (You can also do this just with your husband and other family members as well as with friends or neighbors.)

Benilda Nya

BE FAITHFUL!

Sunday

Cater to your man.

Drink water from your own cistern (container), running water from your own well. Proverbs 5: 15

Monday

Depending on his mood, give him a little sexual appetizer as soon as he gets home.

Tuesday

Wake him up with kisses and whisper, "I am so in love you" in his ear.

Wednesday

Give him a therapeutic massage.

Thursday

Be uncomplicated to love.

Friday

Show him your appreciation… give him a gift with a card inviting him to dinner tomorrow night.

Saturday

Give a dinner party for "two." Look good, cook his favorite dinner and serve it on a well-decorated table (fine linen, china, crystal, candles, favorite wine/beverage and dessert) and play his favorite music. After dessert, surprise him with a relaxing yet sexy bubble bath for "two," or a dip in the hot tub.

NOTES/COMMENTS/JOURNAL: (Keep a record of what worked, changes made or new ideas.)

Daily Coaching – Week 22

Exciting Things to Do Under the Full Moon

❤ Take a few minutes together to gaze at the moon if it is in view and share some romantic thoughts.

❤ Go for an evening stroll arm in arm, around the neighborhood or local park.

❤ If the weather permits have a candle lit dinner in the backyard or balcony under the moonlight.

❤ Rent a limousine, take him out to dinner at an outdoor restaurant with a view of the full moon. Look into his eyes and tell him: "I am so in love with you," talk of sweet and romantic things (be sincere). Kiss and caress him. If possible, get a bit naughty with him in the limo on the way home.

❤ If you have your own private swimming pool, go skinny-dipping and make love to him in the pool.

❤ After dinner, tell him that the moon is full and you want to make the wolf man howl. Turn all the lights off; take him by the hand to a place in the house (that you have prepared with a fur throw) where the moonlight is bright and in view, and proceed with some of his favorites, nice and slow. Use your "sexual romance" arsenal well for this one. You want lots of anticipation on his part. (As always, please provide for privacy.)

Benilda Nya

Choose To Disagree Nicely.

Sunday

Serve him breakfast in bed and give him the day off, let him do nothing if he so wishes.

Better to live on a corner of the roof than share a house with a quarrelsome wife. Proverbs 25: 24

Monday

Wake up counting your blessings; have a happy day!

Tuesday

Make a vision board of your accomplishments.

Wednesday

Have dinner out in your yard, balcony or at the beach.

Thursday

Get rid of procrastination.

Friday

If you have kids you could think about having a family talent show night.

Saturday

Bathe each other in an aromatherapy bubble bath. Light some candles, play some music and have your favorite beverage.

NOTES:

Daily Coaching – Week 23

Make Him Feel Like a Man Should

*M*ost men enjoy seeing the expression in their woman's eyes when they are being made love to. So look at him, talk sexy or make sexy sounds to express your pleasure, let him be the center of your attention. Let your mouth, arms, hands and legs show him how much you enjoy his body. Take your time and do it with passion.

Benilda Nya

You Might Not Be Able To Control The Circumstances, But You Definitely Can Control The Way You React.

Sunday

A wise man/woman has great power, and a man/woman of knowledge increases strength. Proverbs 24: 5

Monday

Make breakfast with great health in mind.

Tuesday

Go out for an evening stroll.

Wednesday

Decide to succeed.

Thursday

Praise him, and tell him that he is very special and precious to you.

Friday

After dinner, go count the stars and watch for falling stars to wish upon.

Saturday

Spend the whole day in bed reading, eating, talking, watching movies, etc.

NOTES/COMMENTS/JOURNAL: (Keep a record of what worked, changes made or new ideas.)

Daily Coaching – Week 24

WARNING – some of the language and suggestions contained below, might be offensive to some.

Pleasure & Excitement

Giving him Sexual Variety will take some desire, know how and effort.

- ❤ What type of outfits does he most like to see you in that sexually arouse him?
- ❤ What type of lighting does he like?
- ❤ What helps him to get into you?
- ❤ How can you dress to turn him on?
- ❤ Are you a good kisser?
- ❤ Do you smell the way he likes?
- ❤ Does he like a sensual massage? Do you know how to give him one?
- ❤ What type of music puts him in the mood?
- ❤ Will satin bed sheets make it more erotic for him?
- ❤ What are his favorites in the foreplay menu?
- ❤ How does he like his after-play?
- ❤ In what places is he most open to make love or have sex?
- ❤ What sexual positions does he like?
- ❤ Let him concentrate on the sensations that you want to provoke in him by you being the giver (do this at least once a month).

Benilda Nya

Be At Peace And Have Faith, While You Are Working To Achieve Your Dreams And Goals. They Will Happen!

Sunday

A heart at peace gives life to the body but envy rots the bones.
Proverbs 14: 30

Monday

Make your dreams a reality by concentrating on the details.

Tuesday

Be confident, think well of yourself and believe in yourself.

Wednesday

Feed your subconscious mind with positive conscious autosuggestions.

Thursday

Play out one of his sexual desires.

Friday

Go ahead and share a piece of string licorice or gum without using your hands.

Saturday

Have breakfast in the backyard or on the porch or balcony.

NOTES:

Daily Coaching – Week 25

Be His #1 Fan

*A*ward your spouse with a plaque or trophy (make it big and/or beautiful) for being "The Greatest" or "Best" _____, or for a professional, sporting or hobby accomplishment. Plan an awards dinner, invite family, friends, co-workers and especially the people that appreciate and respect him and are a part of the group concerning this award. You can send out invitations and make the dinner casual, semi-formal or formal, according to the type of award.

*Y*ou could make it a surprise; just make sure that he is available for that day by asking him for a date or you could just tell him that a dinner is being held in his honor. Let him know how he needs to dress, and lay out his clothes for him. Make sure that he looks good. You could also buy him a new outfit and send him to the barber/salon to get a haircut, shave and manicure.

*S*elect some of these happy supporters to say a few words and make the presentation speech a real good one. You can hold this dinner at his favorite restaurant, sports bar, venue or at home.

Benilda Nya

Develop And Refine Yourself.

Sunday

A quarrelsome wife is like a constant dripping on a rainy day; restraining her is like restraining the wind or grasping oil with the hand. Proverbs 27: 15

Monday

Hello and goodbye kisses are always a delight.

Tuesday

Separate yourself from the people and things that will hinder your success.

Wednesday

Indulge him.

Thursday

Enjoy and welcome his nonsexual romantic approach.

Friday

Look and feel sexy. Have a great loungewear home-line and lingerie arsenal. Use them daily.

Saturday

Go to the beach for a picnic dinner; help him to prepare everything for a beautiful time.

NOTES/COMMENTS/JOURNAL: (Keep a record of what worked, changes made or new ideas.)

Daily Coaching – Week 26

*L*et Him Know that you Treasure Being with Him

💜 When he hugs you or cuddles with you, stay in the present and enjoy his presence, thank him and tell him how much you enjoy that.

💜 Talk if he wants to talk, or simply enjoy silence with him if that's what he wants.

💜 Respect him, and try to understand his frame of mind.

💜 Do not jump to conclusions or misinterpret his words or actions.

💜 Make time for him.

💜 Get to know him so well that just by him looking at you or you looking at him in certain situations, you know what he wants or feels.

💜 Walk hand in hand, arm in arm or with arms around each other.

💜 Hug him for an extensive period of time.

💜 Give him some space, time to himself and time with his friends.

Benilda Nya

Your Most Powerful Tool And Weapon Is YOUR Mouth. Use It Responsibly.

Sunday

The tongue has the power of life and death, and those who love it will eat of its fruit. Proverbs 18: 21

Monday

Learn a new language together.

Tuesday

Praise him for his uniqueness

Wednesday

Until you decide to do it, it's not going to happen.

Thursday

Do some "Pillow" talk.

Friday

Lust after him; undress him with your eyes, and picture yourself doing delicious and sensual things to his body.

Saturday

When he takes you out, dress appropriately for the occasion. Make sure that your hair and makeup are beautiful, and please don't forget to use good social etiquette.

NOTES:

Daily Coaching – Week 27

*L*ook Your Best

DRESS FOR SUCCESS

*Y*our success will depend a lot on your appearance, communication skills (verbal/non-verbal) and business etiquette. Have the right attitude at work and for work.

DRESS SEXY/STYLISH (When You Go Out with Him)

*U*se the right colors and trendy and classic styles to go with your fashion personality and body type. Make sure that your clothes are clean, pressed, fit properly and that you wear them the way the style is supposed to be. Make sure that your clothes are not trashy tight, accentuating any negatives. No split seams, hanging threads, sagging linings or loose buttons. Your shoes should also be clean and polished with no worn out heels and free of bad odors. Under garments should be as new (no holes, stains or tattered).

BE WELL-GROOMED (To guarantee your good looks.)

Hair - Your style should be an updated look that you know how to style between visits to the salon, and it should go with the shape of your face. If you need to color your hair or put highlights in it, make sure that you keep up with the retouching. **Your face** - Use the right products for your skin type. They will keep your skin looking good. Go for a facial at least twice a year. Please make sure that you wear the right makeup colors, and that you know how to apply your makeup properly to bring out your best features. You can also keep up with new make up trends, but only add the colors and shapes that make <u>you</u> look your best. **Facial hair** - Affects your image and beauty, so have it removed. **Eyebrows** - Should be shaped according to the shape of your face and eyes. <u>If you wear eye glasses</u>, wear the right color and shape for your face or get contacts; you can also try to see if laser eye surgery is for you. **Mouth** - Brush & floss daily. Make sure that your breath is fresh. If you have problem or damaged teeth, you can improve their appearance by bleaching, bonding, porcelain veneers or crowns.

Benilda Nya

Success Requires Knowledge.

Sunday

Go to a museum or art gallery.

It is not good to have zeal without knowledge, nor to be hasty and miss the way. Proverbs 19: 2

Monday

Get rid of nagging habits.

Tuesday

Celebrate your beauty.

Wednesday

Always thank him for his thoughtfulness and consideration.

Thursday

Be committed to self-discipline.

Friday

Cuddle after dinner.

Saturday

Take time to relax, talk and listen to each other about any concerns, or plans for something.

NOTES/COMMENTS/JOURNAL: (Keep a record of what worked, changes made or new ideas.)

Daily Coaching – Week 28

Look Your Best - Be Your Best

DRESS FOR SUCCESS

BE WELL-GROOMED (To guarantee your good looks.)

Body - Keep your body clean and your skin soft. Wear the fragrance that he loves on you (lightly). **Body hair** - Underarms, legs, bikini line (if you are hairy, please trim that area as well), abdomen, fingers and hairy arms should be waxed regularly. **<u>Fingernails</u>** - Should be clean and filed with trimmed cuticles, in a length that works for your life-style. Get a manicure and pedicure at least once a month. Perhaps you and your husband can go together to the spa or salon, and make it a "spa" date.

MIND YOUR MANNERS (Use social etiquette)

There is something exceptional about a
woman with good manners.

*Y*our excellent physical appearance and your good manners will open doors, not just in your professional and social life, but in your personal life, as well. Say, "please" and "thank you," when it is fitting. When your husband or someone else opens a door for you, pulls out your chair or pushes the chair in for you, a "thank you" is proper. Have good posture whether sitting or walking (this will also help to keep your body looking young). It is important for you to increase your verbal and non-verbal communication skills. Also, know your dinner etiquette well and use it. Be familiar with the choice of wine or champagne. (It is not fitting to re-apply lipstick or powder your nose at the dinner table.)

MISS CONGENIALITY

*I*t is a pleasure to be around nice people. Be a woman of excellence. Be prudent, use discernment and have integrity, a woman of strength and dignity. When you speak, let your words be wise. To that add self-control and organization, and let them be your guide to success. Be energetic and have a positive outlook about yourself, your marriage, your family, life and people; it will attract a lot of good things to you.

Benilda Nya

Weekly Coaching - Week 29

You Can Only Eat An Elephant One Bite At A Time.

Sunday

Whoever watches the wind will not plant; whoever looks at the clouds will not reap. Ecclesiastes 11: 4

Monday

Encourage and praise his creativity.

Tuesday

Accept his imperfections, and just concentrate on his strengths.

Wednesday

Your happiness does not depend on him, but it is for you to create.

Thursday

Ask him if there is anything that he needs your help with to achieve his goals.

Friday

Never take for granted or get dispassionate about him giving you gifts, flowers and showing his love and appreciation to you.

Saturday

Ride a bicycle built for two.

NOTES:

Daily Coaching – Week 29

Be Your Best
AT HOME

*W*ear beautiful or sexy loungewear; try to look your best even at home. Keep your home clean, neat, and smelling good, with a peaceful atmosphere. The way you keep your home is a reflection of your spirit and soul. Even your yard (front and back) or balcony reflects your personality. Your home is your castle, so make it a beautiful and pleasant place to live in. Watch carefully all that goes on throughout your household, and never be lazy. Get up early to prepare breakfast. If you have a maid, plan the day's work for her. Whether you work outside of the home or at home, make sure that a good dinner is always served. You or your husband can prepare the food the night before so that who ever gets home first can start to cook dinner.

COMMUNITY LIAISON

*G*et involved in your community; vote and volunteer to help in community projects (but do not over-do it and neglect your home). Help those in need, feed the hungry, clothed the naked, help the fatherless and widows. Be a good neighbor. Become a mentor. Join a good church or synagogue.

FINANCIALLY SAVVY

*C*heap things are never good, so watch for bargains to make your purchases. Plan the budget with your husband and stick to it. Use those coupons, and get those rebates. Shop smart. Learn to manage your money by diligently tracking your spending. Make informed financial decisions.

SELF HELP

*R*echarge, refuel and relax yourself. Do not just give and give of yourself without giving yourself time to replenish your spirit, soul and body. Get yourself a mentor or two. Learn to discern who is a friend and who is an acquaintance, or who is a work buddy or just a fellow employee. Use wisdom and self-control in what you say and how much you say and to whom. Choose to be happy, and to be grateful.

Benilda Nya

Weekly Coaching - Week 30

What You Do Daily Will Determine Your Future.

Sunday

Lazy hands make a man poor, but diligent hands brings wealth.
Proverbs 10: 4

Monday

Take a walk hand in hand or go for a drive after dinner.

Tuesday

Take a shower with him.

Wednesday

WARNING: use only if appropriate for both of you. Make love in a different place: the backyard, balcony, at the beach, at the park, in the car, on your boat/yacht. Please make sure that you have privacy.

Thursday

Preparation is the key to handling the opportunities and obstacles along the way.

Friday

Have a candle light dinner in the backyard or balcony.

Saturday

Read to one another in bed.

NOTES/COMMENTS/JOURNAL: (Keep a record of what worked, changes made or new ideas.)

Daily Coaching – Week 30

There's always a reason to Celebrate!

❤ *H*ow do you feel when you celebrate? Do you get happy and full of enthusiasm? Then you should copy this euphoric feeling as often as possible.

❤ *T*hrow a party to celebrate yourself, your husband, your marriage, and your loved ones or just to simply rejoice about life itself. Celebrate this beautiful planet that God created for you to get pleasure from, because He wants you to live your life with significance and determination.

Benilda Nya

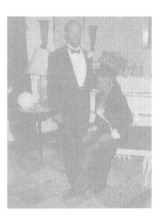

(Place a picture here of you and your spouse at a party.)

With Prosperity Comes The Responsibility Of Purpose.

Sunday

The Lord will send a blessing on your barns and on everything you put your hand to. The Lord your God will bless you in the land He is giving you. Deuteronomy 28: 8

Monday

Show him and tell him how much you value him.

Tuesday

After dinner, do some cheek-to-cheek dancing by candlelight.

Wednesday

Gladly do what he asks you to do.

Thursday

Get good at forgiving, because people will always disappoint you.

Friday

Set the table beautifully for dinner, candles and all.

Saturday

Give a beach party with your husband for your friends and relatives.

NOTES:

Daily Coaching – Week 31

*E*ncourage him to share his sexual fantasies with you and whenever possible, surprise him by playing the lead and making it happen. Whatever it might be, do not make him feel weird or silly for sharing; just play with the ones that you are comfortable with and/or arouse you.

Benilda Nya

Don't Just Exist ... Live Everyday With Purpose And Reach Your Potential.

Sunday

...then nothing they plan to do will be impossible for them. Genesis 11: 6

Monday

Wake him up by kissing and caressing him, and then make love to him.

Tuesday

Take time out for fun and games.

Wednesday

Go for a walk with arms around each other, and tell him that he's an awesome man.

Thursday

Be friendly and fun to be with.

Friday

Go to bed naked.

Saturday

Go out for breakfast. Afterwards go to the park and go boating and/ or horseback riding. If it is possible, make out with him on the boat or a private spot somewhere in the park.

NOTES/COMMENTS/JOURNAL: (Keep a record of what worked, changes made or new ideas.)

Daily Coaching – Week 32

Honor Him

Tell him how valuable he is to you.

. . . .

Love him by sacrificing for him.

. . . .

Work out the disagreements.

. . . .

Make him your top priority.

. . . .

Be willing to do for him.

. . . .

Be committed to him.

. . . .

Be his best friend.

Benilda Nya

When You Give To Help Those In Need, You Open The Doors For Wonderful Things To Come To You.

Sunday

A generous man will prosper; he who refreshes others will himself be refreshed. Proverbs 11: 25

Monday

Float together in the pool, or go for a night swim.

Tuesday

Do not get bored with the daily practice of fundamentals.

Wednesday

Whenever he takes you away for the weekend or does something extraordinary, send him an arrangement of his favorite flowers or a gift to his job with a thank you card.

Thursday

Dedicate a song to him on his favorite radio station (make sure he is listening).

Friday

Be attentive to his needs and wants.

Saturday

Wine and dine, reminisce together; create some new memories.

NOTES:

Daily Coaching – Week 33

Love Notes

- Send him an erotic dinner or lunch invitation: "Sexy Chef" will be cooking up an erogenous five course meal, on ____. "Minimum" attire required.
- Next time you are cooking a romantic dinner for him make a menu and describe each item on the menu in a very sexy and erotic way.
- Write a sensual poem on beautiful parchment paper describing how he makes you feel, kiss his name at the beginning (your lips imprinted with his favorite color lipstick, write his name between the lips). Spray it with his favorite perfume, scroll it and tie with a ribbon. Place it on a small decorative pillow (a royalty look), and hand it to him as you bow.
- Leave little stick-ums with kisses (your lips imprinted with lipstick) in places where he can find them and write sweet little nothings on them.
- Write him a thank you note (for something special he did, etc.), or send him a card or letter to tell him how proud you are of him.
- Send him a formal invite with an RSVP the next time you want to give him an extraordinary surprise.
- Send him the appropriate color roses/flowers with the coordinating love note. For example: Assorted color roses together with a note that says... "You're everything to me."
- Make him his own personal "girly" calendar. Do a variety of poses: sexy, erotic, sweet (make sure your eyes talk to him). Purchase a calendar program for your computer, then take the twelve best pictures and create the calendar. With a scanner and printer you can create it yourself. Use your own camera and safe guard your pictures. You can also make this a "photo shoot date" and take pictures of each other to create the calendars together (make one of him too). Great foreplay!

Search in the Bible for "The Song of Solomon" (second book after Proverbs); it is full of sexy and beautiful poems that you can use. Go to the Library or bookstore and find books that can help you write poems and love letters.

Benilda Nya

Get Wisdom.

Sunday

Blessed is the man/woman who finds wisdom, and the man/woman who gains understanding. Proverbs 3: 13

Monday

Keep him madly in love.

Tuesday

Give him a compliment daily. Be specific.

Wednesday

When he shows you affection, tell him: "you make my fairy tales come true."

Thursday

With practice, you can make yourself happier.

Friday

Enrich your relationship; tell him "I love you."

Saturday

Have a captivating attitude with him.

NOTES/COMMENTS/JOURNAL: (Keep a record of what worked, changes made or new ideas.)

Daily Coaching – Week 34

$\mathcal{B}$uild and/or Decorate Your House
With Romance in Mind

- **Overall Design:** large windows, arched doorways, high ceilings, split levels, columns, sky lights, sky lights, atriums and spacious rooms. Beautiful doors and hardware. Water fountain.
- **Living room:** columns, arched doorways, tray ceiling, wall water fall/fountain. Silk or chiffon/sheer drapes. Shaggy rug, wood, marble or glass tile flooring with a shaggy area rug.
- **Family room:** fireplace, silk/chiffon/velvet drapes.
- **Game Room/Area:** velvet drapes, pool table, card & board games, ping-pong or hockey table and video games.
- **Media Room:** surround sound screen T.V. Fluffy oversized leather (or other soft fabric) sofa, oversized reclining chairs and a center table/ottoman.
- **Library:** leather wing chairs and sofa, floor-to-ceiling built in mahogany bookshelves and a computer station.
- **Master Bedroom:** fireplace, top of the line mattress and four poster/canopy bed, decorative iron or upholstered headboard with fabric draping from the ceiling to the floor. Chandelier above the bed, if possible, or wall lighting sconces for soft lighting; scented candles. Fresh roses/flowers, crisp or silky linen, and if there is room for a sitting area, create a sensual setting with extra large decorative pillows, a furry floor rug and a low upholstered coffee table. And a stereo to play some of that romantic music you have.
- **Master Bathroom:** shower built for two with multiple shower heads and a built-in seat. Roman/Jacuzzi tub built for two with air jets and heater. chandelier, curtains and aromatic candles are a must.
- **Dining Room:** with beautiful furniture, columns; chandelier, and trim the windows with silk or chiffon drapes.
- **Your Balcony:** can also be a nest for "romance" depending on where and how it is facing. You can put plants, torches, a hammock, white outdoor curtains, patio furniture or add a café table so that you may enjoy eating outside.

$\mathcal{B}$enilda $\mathcal{N}$ya

How Are You Handling The Difficult Things In Life?
Your Children Are Watching And Learning.

Sunday

Children's children are a crown to the aged, and parents are the pride of their children. Proverbs 17: 6

Monday

See the "challenge" in a trial not the burden.

Tuesday

Bake his favorite cake or pie.

Wednesday

Improve your sex appeal.

Thursday

Be proud of your body.

Friday

Have a cheerful attitude.

Saturday

Have an emotional interaction…share deep feelings.

NOTES:

Daily Coaching – Week 35

- ❤ **Backyard:** landscape with security and privacy in mind. You'll need it to be able to enjoy "romantic" moments in the swimming pool or hot tub. You can also build or buy a pond with a waterfall design and fill it with water plants and gold fish. Create a beautiful and romantic area for eating outdoors. Build a cabana, loggia, sitting and/or lounging area with a theme: Moroccan, Roman, Spanish, Jungle look, etc. Install a beautiful birdbath and plant flowers that will attract butterflies and humming birds. If possible, have an outdoor sound system (be considerate of your neighbors, keep the volume low to moderate).

- ❤ **Party Room:** design a sound proof room where you can build a small stage with stage lighting. Maybe add a sliding pole, curtains and a nice backdrop. Have a beverage area/bar with stools. For sitting, use low, upholstered platforms topped with extra big decorative pillows. Trim the walls with mirrors, the windows with ceiling to floor curtains, low center tables and soft lighting. The sound system should be well equipped with the best music of every category that you both enjoy, especially romantic music. I'm sure you, your spouse and children (if any) can use that stage for private or family performances.

- ❤ **In your car:** keep a "love basket" equipped with a towel, blanket, etcetera. Whether in the car, on the beach, at the park or your favorite scenic view, you can be prepared for those planned or spontaneous "romantic" encounters with your husband.

- ❤ **If you rent:** you can still decorate your place to be really romantic by the size and shape of your furniture and the fabrics that you choose. Have floor-to-ceiling drapes, a framed mirror in the dining room, candles, wall sconces/stands, candles in the bathroom, and bedroom. Accent with throw rugs, decorative pillows, fresh flowers and your favorite scents. A great sound system is a must for your favorite music (be considerate of your neighbors, keep the volume low to moderate).

A clean and well-organized home is always a plus when it comes to enriching the "romantic" atmosphere in your home. The house should always have fresh flowers and in-door plants, candles, or maybe even a water fountain and your house should smell great.

Benilda Nya

Wisdom Has Great Benefits.

Sunday

Wisdom will prolong your life many years and bring you prosperity. The wise inherit honor. Proverbs 3: 2, 35

Monday

Indulge the senses, and prepare a seductive meal.

Tuesday

Call him during the day and ask him out on a date for Friday. Take him out to one of his favorite places and treat him like the king that he is by paying for everything. Lay out the clothes that you want him to wear. If possible, rent the fancy sports car that he likes, and have him drive it.

Wednesday

Wake him up with kisses and if time permits, serve him breakfast in bed.

Thursday

Show him lots of appreciation.

Friday

Have a happy time treating him like the king that he is.

Saturday

Enjoy your well-deserved pampering.

NOTES/COMMENTS/JOURNAL: (Keep a record of what worked, changes made or new ideas.)

Daily Coaching – Week 36

$\mathcal{P}$ut on your Marriage Armor

(So that you can stand against the schemes that lead to betrayal & divorce.)

❤ **Belt of Truth:** you love your mate that is why you chose him. Ask him (with the right attitude, at a time of intimacy) for what you need that he might not be giving you, instead of trying to find it in someone or something else. Spend quality time together with your mate. Nurture your relationship with him; do not get wrapped up into working so hard to make ends meet or being an overachiever that you neglect your home and his needs. You and your family will suffer the consequences, so please find a good balance.

❤ **Breastplate:** safeguard against spending time with the wrong people (a woman that is not interested in the sanctity of marriage or that might disrespect your husband or children or a man that you might find interesting or attractive). Avoid spending private time with other men, and you must watch what you talk about with other men; it should not be anything that is intimate or sexual because these subjects have been known to start a sexual relationship, even between people who where not looking to go astray or found each other interesting or attractive. That is another reason why being intimate with your mate is imperative for a healthy relationship.

❤ **Feet built-in:** be ready to immediately walk away from the circumstances that will be detrimental for your marriage, your personal and professional life. Do not look for the wrong things to fill any voids in your marriage.

Benilda Nya

Visualize And Plan Your Perfect Week.

Sunday

The plans of the diligent lead to profit... Proverbs 21: 5

Monday

See if you can take him out to lunch.

Tuesday

Give him soft kisses on his face, eyes, nose, neck and shoulders while he's watching TV.

Wednesday

Have peace and faith in the midst of trials.

Thursday

Show him and tell him how much you admire him.

Friday

Enhance your relationship; tell him "I am so in love with you."

Saturday

Empower yourself with courage to do the things that you know you must do, even though you may not want to do them.

NOTES:

Daily Coaching – Week 37

*P*ut on your Marriage Armor

(So that you can stand against the schemes that lead to betrayal & divorce.)

💜 **Shield:** have faith in God, yourself and in your mate for a successful relationship. This faith will put out those flaming arrows that will attack you and try to sabotage your integrity, your present and your future. Pray for your marriage and family daily.

💜 **Helmet:** protect your eyes; control your mind and your thoughts. What you think about and visualize is what will happen. (If you see that the grass looks greener on the other side, it is only because somebody was willing to nurture, fertilize, water and pull out the weeds, or it's a facade.)

💜 **Sword:** intimacy, sexual and verbal communication. Focus on the attention needed to fulfill one another. Your marriage is not just a fifty/fifty effort, but it is for both of you to give a hundred percent, even two-hundred percent or more.

Benilda Nya

BREATHE In Deeply, Exhale Slowly, And THINK Before You Speak.

Sunday

A gentle answer turns away wrath, but a harsh word stirs up anger.

Proverbs 15: 1

Monday

Enjoy his kisses and him caressing you at the movies.

Tuesday

Renew your mind (the way you perceive things).

Wednesday

Keep the home fire burning hot, hotter and hottest!

Thursday

Greet him with a big kiss and hug and say to him: "I've been waiting all day long for this moment."

Friday

In certain things, be and act independent; do not be a needy or high maintenance woman.

Saturday

Make plans to take a vacation at a very romantic place.

NOTES/COMMENTS/JOURNAL: (Keep a record of what worked, changes made or new ideas.)

Daily Coaching – Week 38

When he gets home tired from work...

💜 **S**urprise him with a nice hot bath with his favorite oil scent and a long back or full body massage (15-30 minutes), to put him to sleep with.

💜 **S**urprise him with a luxurious, hot foot soak with Epsom salt and his favorite scented oil, followed by a foot massage; especially if he worked on his feet all day.

💜 **S**urprise him with some peace and quiet. Give him some time to un-wind from his day. Ask him if he would like something to drink or eat, then after you give him what he requested, kiss him and tell him to call you if he needs anything. Then quietly go do what you need to do. If you have children/teenagers, go take them for a walk, the park or video games arcade for about an hour.

💜 **S**urprise him when he comes back home from a business trip; pick him up in a limo, look sexy and smell the way he loves. Find out ahead of time what he would like to eat, and have it ready for him to eat with his favorite beverage, and eat and drink on the drive home (make sure that the driver takes his time and maybe even take the scenic view drive).

Benilda Nya

Check And Double Check Your Motives.

Sunday

All a man's ways seem innocent to him, but motives are weighed by the Lord. Proverbs 16: 2

Monday

Be his wife, not his Mother; leave the mothering to his mother.

Tuesday

Tell him that he is very handsome.

Wednesday

Work and play at being romantic.

Thursday

Order dinner from one of his favorite restaurants.

Friday

Have a good and vast selection of games to play. You can also buy a karaoke machine and sing to each other.

Saturday

Great sex starts in your head, so prepare your mind to get physically in the mood. Start with your touch. The way you touch and caress him will draw out and transmit sexual expression from both of you. Your hands are an excellent source for pleasure.

NOTES:

Daily Coaching – Week 39

A **Mighty Fortress**

❤ **F**rom the landscaping and the lighting outside of the house to the doors and windows and the inside of the house, make sure that your home is well-protected against intruders. Have an alarm that can function even if the phone lines are cut.

❤ **W**hen at home, the windows and doors should have a chime to let you know if they are opened.

❤ **I**f he is going out of town and you are staying home, make sure that all safety devices are working and use them.

❤ **C**reate a safety room in the house, or a way out in case of fire or danger.

Benilda Nya

Sow Seeds Of Kindness... Be Kind To Yourself And Others.

Sunday

A kind man/woman benefits him/her self, but a cruel man brings trouble on himself. Proverbs 11: 17

Monday

Respect yourself, so that others can also respect you.

Tuesday

Before he goes to work, make him a healthy lunch, pack it up, and put a love note inside the bag.

Wednesday

Wake him up with your soft caressing and kissing.

Thursday

Romantic love is exclusive for your lifetime commitment.

Friday

Have an inspiring conversation with him, and create excitement with your tone of voice.

Saturday

Prepare a nice and hot aromatherapy bubble bath for the two of you and talk about your dreams and goals. (Serve his and your favorite beverage and snacks.)

NOTES/COMMENTS/JOURNAL: (Keep a record of what worked, changes made or new ideas.)

Daily Coaching – Week 40

A Safe Haven

♥ **T**he car should also have an alarm and a prompt recovery device.

♥ **Y**ou should carry some type of protection in your purse.

♥ **T**ake some form of personal protection class; you can make it a family time event.

♥ **M**ake your home a "green" home. Buy organic/natural as much as possible: foods, personal hygiene products, hair and skin care products, cosmetics, household cleaners, bedding, furnishings and accessories. Improve the quality of your water by using a filtration system, and an air purifying system will give you and your family better air to breath. You can also buy indoor plants that help clean the air inside your home. When painting and/or remodeling the house use organic/non-toxic paints and supplies. You can also improve the air inside your car with an Auto Ionizer.

Benilda Nya

To Increase Your Chances For An Excellent And Healthy Life; Help Each Other To Fulfill Your Hopes And Dreams.

Sunday

Go out for brunch and afterwards go ice-skating; hold hands while skating

Hope deferred (postponed/delayed) makes the heart sick, but a longing fulfilled is a tree of life. Proverbs 13: 12

Monday

Improve your problem solving skills.

Tuesday

Make his favorite dinner; serve it on your fine china; serve the wine in your crystal.

Wednesday

Call him at work, and ask him out on a date for Saturday.

Have a movie night at home, cover yourselves with a blanket and cuddle as you watch the movie.

Thursday

Fondle him back when he fondles you.

Friday

Life is not perfect, people are not perfect, relationships are not perfect, so do not expect perfection. People and circumstances will disappoint you, so just learn from the mistakes and try to see the good that can come from the experience; always do your best to look for the decent qualities in people

Saturday

Take him out to his favorite restaurant or sports bar.

NOTES:

Daily Coaching – Week 41

117

His Comfort

❤ **I**f you drive, even if he takes care of the car, you still should know how to keep it well maintained. Learn how to check the oils, the battery and how to change a flat (make sure that all the tools and the spare tire are there and in proper shape). Also learn how to maintain your bicycle, if you have one.

❤ **T**hese days a cell phone is no longer a luxury, but a necessity. Make sure you both have one and, if the children are old enough, they too, should have one. You can also invest in a satellite phone just incase you need one.

❤ **L**et him take pleasure in protecting you, the kids, your home and car. Praise him for it, and you can reward your "Knight in Shining Armor" with a little "*frolicking*" around the fortress.

Benilda Nya

With The Proper Balance, Work Hard For Your Marriage And Your Career.

Sunday

Cook his favorite breakfast foods and yours, and have breakfast in bed.
All hard work brings a profit… Proverbs 14: 23

Monday

Continue to polish your plans; strive for excellence.

Tuesday

Surprise him with a gift after breakfast.

Wednesday

Make love to him or let him do what he wants to you. Keep the lights on (use soft lighting – rose or coral).

Thursday

Celebrate your accomplishments.

Friday

Whenever it applies, tell him that he is physically strong.

Saturday

Kiss him, hug him, squeeze him and please him.

If he is going away on a business trip, make some real good, long love to him the night before, or if possible, in the morning of the day that he is leaving. Pack his clothes for him, and also pack the panties that he loves to see on you. Spray it with your signature fragrance; put it in a plastic sandwich bag with an erotic love note or sexy audiotape/CD, or make a music video where you are the one singing (karaoke or make believe), or dancing.

NOTES/COMMENTS/JOURNAL: (Keep a record of what worked, changes made or new ideas.)

Daily Coaching – Week 42

Forever Exciting Him
10 Commandments

1. Cultivate your marriage with words: "I'm in love with you." "Thank you." "Please." How can I help? "I appreciate you." "I was wrong." "I'm sorry." "I forgive you." "I can't imagine my life without you." "You are so handsome." "I love it when you _____." etc.

2. Communicate, Connect and Listen: be honest about your feelings, share your thoughts and dreams/goals, help him to understand you. Listen to him, encourage and understand him. Be patient; talk about decisions together. It takes time to develop a meaningful communication. Look at conflicts as the doorway to better intimacy and wisdom, so deal with them openly and directly.

3. Be physical and passionate: hug, kiss, caress & flirt. Celebrate and praise him, contribute in all duties, aim to please him, look your best.

4. Lead by your actions: set a good example; plant what you want to harvest; if you want more and lasting success – pray daily and if possible include your husband and family.

5. Give your mate the freedom to think for himself: his originality and intelligence will increase your own. Relax, do not require for your mate and children to act exactly like you and do things the way that you do.

6. There is no place for: unresolved anger, manipulation and harsh criticism.

7. Be fun to live with.

8. Live beyond the blame game.

9. Make deposits: have a positive attitude, lend an ear, a helping hand, non-sexual romance, thoughtfulness, kindness. **Not withdrawals:** Being unappreciative, selfish, negative words and attitude, unkind, unreliable.

10. As much as possible, position your spouse to receive the best first: by doing that you will create a marriage that surpasses all wedding-day dreams, where love not only lasts, but it grows constantly. The honeymoon is on a continual basis.

Benilda Nya

What Is Your Face Saying About You?

Sunday

A happy heart makes the face cheerful, but heartache crushes the spirit.

Proverbs 15: 13

Monday

Handle money the right way.

Tuesday

Look into his eyes when you talk to him about your day.

Wednesday

You have the right to have pleasure… get a bit naughty with him.

Thursday

Smile and be happy; feel like the fabulous hot woman that you are.

Friday

Be interested in what he likes to do: sports, hobbies, his work etc.

Saturday

Be open and transparent with each other.

NOTES:

Daily Coaching - Week 43

The Ordinary vs. the Extraordinary Life

The Ordinary Life (The Basics)

Work, cook, clean, do the laundry, pay the rent/mortgage, pay the bills and car payment(s), groceries, replenishing clothes and shoes. Going to the beauty salon once or twice a month, sex once a week. The expected gifts: Birthday, Valentine's, Anniversary, Father's Day, Christmas, and Hanukkah. Leisure: movies, dinner, etc. once or twice a month, home furnishings.

The Extraordinary Life

- ❤ **Work:** whether you work at home, have your own business or work for somebody else, you are happy to do what you do and you do it with excellence and integrity.

- ❤ **Cooking:** your husband (and kids, if any) should always have healthy and delicious meals to eat at home. Your husband should never come home after a day's work to find no dinner ready, unless the plans are to eat out. A healthy breakfast is also a must.

- ❤ **Clean:** your house, your business and even the car(s). Always keep them clean, neat and well-organized. With his approval or if your budget allows it; hire a maid to clean and a trusted handyman to fix things around the house.

- ❤ **Do the laundry:** never allow the dirty clothes to pile up. Everything should be pressed (you, your husband and kids should never go out with wrinkled clothes), and whatever needs to be sent to the cleaners is sent. Your closets and drawers are also well-organized. If you want your husband to be considered for that promotion and increase your financial status, then you should want to make sure that he always looks the part: well-dressed and groomed.

Benilda Nya

Your Words And Your Actions; Will Build Or Destroy.

Sunday

The wise woman builds/develops her house… The foolish one tears hers down. Proverbs 14: 1

Monday

Never get tired of going out of your way to please and excite him.

Tuesday

Use your body language to flirt with him, talk sexy and drive him wild.

Wednesday

Do not crowd him; give him his space.

Thursday

Use common sense.

Friday

Take your creativity to the next level… Serve dinner while wearing boots, a fur bikini and hat.

Saturday

Go to the park for a carriage ride.

NOTES/COMMENTS/JOURNAL: (Keep a record of what worked, changes made or new ideas.)

Daily Coaching – Week 44

The Extraordinary Life

❤ **Bills/Finances:** pay the rent/mortgage, the bills and car payment(s): before the due date. Pay the full amount you spent on your credit cards, or pay double or triple the minimum payment due. Pay two or more car or mortgage payments whenever possible.

❤ **Groceries:** when you go grocery-shopping buy the best and the healthiest foods. Buy your husband and children (if any) their favorite foods to eat, as well as the favorite brands of toiletries and cleaning items.

❤ **Replenishing clothes and shoes:** shop other than just when needed, according to the budget that you and your spouse have agreed upon.

❤ **Going to the beauty salon:** if the budget does not stretch for regular visits to the salon, then learn how to maintain the look until the next visit.

❤ **Intimacy:** living a life of non-sexual romance, and pleasurable sexual romance (sex in a variety of places and ways), more than once a week. Wear pretty loungewear around the house and pretty or sexy lingerie every day. Have a variety of sleep wear: pretty, feminine, sexy, erotic, long/short, in his and your favorite colors (during your monthly time, you can still look nice because it will help you feel better).

Get Rid Of Your Negative Emotions.

Sunday

Each heart knows its own bitterness, and no one else can share its joy.
Proverbs 14: 10

Monday

Be grateful for the way that he honors you.

Tuesday

Place your favorite bed cover on the couch, and invite him over for some amazing sex in wild positions.

Wednesday

Use your brain properly: envision yourself acting and responding to stressful or negative situations and people the proper way. By doing this, you will learn to change your mind.

Thursday

Avoid negative criticism; be understanding, loving and sincere.

Friday

Have dinner and dessert in bed, surrounded by candlelight, and talk about your first date

Saturday

Be happy to experience life together.

NOTES:

Daily Coaching – Week 45

The Extraordinary Life

♥ **Gifts:** make it a "Birthday," "Anniversary," "Valentine's," "Father's Day," month. Send him flowers or buy him something that you know he wants. Give him gifts to; thank him, praise him, congratulate him or to motivate him. You can also give him a naughty gift to flirt with him.

♥ **Leisure:** depending on your budget, you can do a variety of things on a weekly basis.

♥ **Home furnishings:** should never be worn out or broken. Keep a beautifully furnished home; you can do this even on a tight budget. Let your husband know about things that need replacing or fixing.

Everything that you do for him and with him should have a very special touch. Go that extra mile to please your spouse just because you enjoy making him happy and you delight in showing your love, appreciation and respect for him. You should be devoted to and concerned about the things that are important to him. When your aim is to please him, that's when you'll know that you are giving him an extraordinary and excellent marriage.

Benilda Nya

Be Careful With What You Allow To Enter You.

Sunday

Hold on to instruction, do not let it go; guard it well, for it is your life. Proverbs 4: 13

Monday

Respond instead of reacting.

Tuesday

Keep on getting better; keep improving yourself and your techniques.

Wednesday

Call him and ask him out to lunch. Talk about pleasant things. Flirt with him.

Thursday

You can't change each other, but if you give and take, and appreciate him, your lives will go a lot smoother.

Friday

Build him up in accordance with his need.

Saturday

Honor your love for him: give him a kiss if you are the one who is right in a discussion or disagreement.

NOTES/COMMENTS/JOURNAL: (Keep a record of what worked, changes made or new ideas.)

Daily Coaching—Week 46

Have Dinner Cabaret style

Have dinner "Chicago" style (the musical). Cook or order the type of food that is served in a cabaret, serve the type of drink that he would order; sing and dance for him.

Set up an area decorated cabaret style. Have music playing, dress like a cabaret waitress, and serve him a couple of drinks. Then slip away to quickly change into an outfit like in the movie; play the song you liked the best, and sing and dance along with it. Have fun!

Benilda Nya

RESPECT Your Money.

Sunday

Cook his favorite foods, including the ones that his mother made for him when he lived with her.

Dishonest money dwindles away, but he who gathers money little by little makes it grow. Proverbs 13: 11

Monday

Accompany each other to doctor/dentist appointments.

Tuesday

On a cold morning or night, warm up his terry cloth slippers, robe and his towel; hand them to him after his shower.

Wednesday

Excite him… Be his Geisha girl tonight.

Thursday

Talk about the visions you share.

Friday

When he takes you away, undress in front of him. Make sure you're wearing sexy underwear.

Saturday

Do the little things, they count too.

Pick a night next week when you can sit down with your husband (and older children, if any). Take pen and paper, and design the way that you want your new year to be. Write down your wants, needs, dreams, goals and the steps that need to be taken to accomplish these dreams and goals. Decide to create the right attitude by making the choices that will take you there.

NOTES:

Daily Coaching – Week 47

*Y*ou and your spouse should work on creating an excellent atmosphere in your home, so that your home is one of the best and safest places; a lifeline that you can cling to to increase peace and joy, a place where you are able to de-stress and get away from the not so great things and people in your day. Your home should be your castle, your hiding place and sanctuary. It should be a place for rejuvenation; make your home your spa away from the spa. Let yourself be these things for your mate and children, as well.

*T*ake time out every day to de-brief, so that you can prevent burnout. *Choose* to encourage yourself for improving the quality of your marriage/relationship and thus, refining the quality of your life.

*L*ife is about choices. So choose to love yourself and others; choose to be happy and to have integrity; choose peace and excellence. These things will only help you to reach your goals and to live the life you dream of.

Benilda Nya

Pursue Wisdom.

Sunday

The wisdom of the prudent is to give thought to their ways… Proverbs 14: 8

Monday

Pinch or grab his buns, kiss him and tell him that he looks good enough to eat.

Tuesday

Tell him, "I love you" in Spanish… "Te Amo." (See page 218 for saying "I love you" in other languages)

Wednesday

Praise and thank him for being thoughtful and helpful.

Thursday

Persist in the pursuit of a "blissful" marriage; it is achievable.

Friday

Learn about your spouse's character (nature, disposition, tendencies).

Saturday

Tuck him in, kiss him and give him a hand massage.

NOTES/COMMENTS/JOURNAL: (Keep a record of what worked, changes made or new ideas.)

Daily Coaching – Week 48

*N*ow *It's the Time!*

*E*njoy where you are at while on the way to where you are going

....

*S*top to smell the roses

....

*B*e aware of all the beautiful things around you

....

*Y*ou have the power to make everyday an extraordinary day

Benilda Nya

*K*eep Moving Forward!

*C*heck your mental vision; make sure that it is not distorted

....

*S*top functioning in your dysfunction

....

*Y*our past does not have to determine your future

....

*T*alk about yourself the way that you imagine yourself to be/how you want to be

....

*Y*ou yourself are a miracle and can make miracles happen; so never stop hoping, believing, praying and giving and doing your best

Benilda Nya

Weekly Coaching

For the next four weeks, I want you to create the daily Non-Sexual and Sexual Romance ideas that your mate will love for you to carry out. I am sure that you will do an excellent job and enjoy doing it.

Sow Seeds Of Kindness... Be Kind To Yourself And Others.

Sunday

A kind man/woman benefits him/herself, but a cruel man brings trouble on him/herself. Proverbs 11: 17

Monday

Tuesday

Wednesday

Thursday

Friday

Saturday

NOTES:

Daily Coaching – Week 49

Weekly Coaching - Week 50

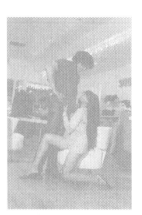

(Place a picture of both of you here.)

You Were Created To Succeed.

Sunday

A faithful man/woman will be richly blessed. Proverbs 28: 20

Monday

Tuesday

Wednesday

Thursday

Friday

Saturday

NOTES/COMMENTS/JOURNAL: (Keep a record of what worked, changes made or new ideas.)

Daily Coaching – Week 50

Communication Advice From A Licensed Counselor

*C*ommunication in a relationship is crucial. Many couples fail to see the importance of their communication. When couples communicate effectively, they are able to understand each other better. Communication is a shared responsibility because it is a way of defining ourselves to our partner. It does not matter how old you are or how long you have been in your relationship, you still need to learn how to communicate your feelings and emotions to your partner. Your communication should be open and honest. It should not be used to create shame or guilt or ridiculing. An open and honest relationship with caring and sympathy is the key to a successful relationship.

An effective and warm listener can be a key to resolving conflicts when the relationship is failing. Communicating like "true friends" can enhance the time spent together. Couples need to find time alone, sit down together and discuss their concerns with each other more often than they do. When couples don't take the time to do this on a regular basis, other less effective ways of communicating such as gestures, tone of voice, anger, silence and rejection can become a normal part of your communication process. These means of communication are not only hurtful, but they also act as a barrier to building a strong relationship.

It is not a healthy manner of communicating to each other, but it sends a clear message to your partner that someone is not happy about something and chooses not to openly discuss the problem with his/her partner. It is sometimes a good idea to write a letter to your partner and try to be as open and honest as you can possibly be. Tell him/her how you feel. This is a good way of starting a conversation and to effectively convey a clear message to your partner that you do not want to continue feeling upset about something. The other partner's interpretation can be enhanced by asking questions and becoming an empathetic listener. It is sometimes difficult to have couples attentively listen without interrupting the other partner or becoming defensive. Keeping an open and non-judge mental attitude can help you build a more positive relationship. Maintaining open doors for more discussions can be another avenue to restart a conversation in the near future.

Become A Better You... Confront And Conquer Your Problems With A Positive Mental Attitude.

Sunday

...The desires of the diligent are fully satisfied. Proverbs 13: 4

....

Monday

....

Tuesday

....

Wednesday

....

Thursday

....

Friday

....

Saturday

NOTES/COMMENTS/JOURNAL: (Keep a record of what worked, changes made or new ideas.)

We all need to be aware that our personal communication style may need to be enhanced. We may need to search ourselves first and make a personal inventory before we can understand our partner. Don't be afraid to research books and to educate yourself in how to become an effective listener and communicator. This will not only enhance your relationship with your partner, but it will enhance your relationship with your children and others in your life.

Article written by: Maritza Montano, PhD
Licensed Mental Health Counselor
Board Certified Counselor
Diplomat of American Psychotherapist Association

If you would like more information regarding this topic, you can E-Mail Dr. Montano at: MLStres1@bellsouth.net

Motivate Yourself With A Positive Mental Attitude And You Will Also Motivate Your Mate And those Around You.

Sunday

A cheerful look brings joy to the heart, and good news gives health to the bones. Proverbs 11: 17

Monday

Tuesday

Wednesday

Thursday

Friday

Saturday

NOTES:

Daily Coaching – Week 52

Warning Against Adultery

*M*y son, pay attention to my wisdom, listen well to my words of insight, that you may maintain discretion and your lips may preserve knowledge. For the lips of an adulteress drip honey, and her speech is smoother than oil; but in the end she is bitter as gall, sharp as a double-edged sword. Her feet go down to death; her steps lead straight to the grave. She gives no thought to the way of life; her paths are crooked, but she knows it not.

Now then, my sons, listen to me; do not turn aside from what I say. Keep to a path far from her, do not go near the door of her house, lest you give your best strength to others and your years to one who is cruel, lest strangers feast on your wealth and your toil enrich another man's house. At the end of your life you will groan, when your flesh and body are spent. You will say, "How I hated discipline! How my heart spurned correction! I would not obey my teachers or listen to my instructors. I have come to the brink of utter ruin in the midst of the whole assembly."

Drink water from your own cistern, running water from your own well. Should your springs overflow in the streets, your streams of water in the public squares? Let them be yours alone, never to be shared with strangers. May your fountain be blessed, and may you rejoice in the Wife of your youth. A loving doe, a graceful deer may her breasts satisfy you always, may you ever be captivated by her love. Why be captivated, my son, by an adulteress?

Why embrace the bosom of another man's wife?

For a man's ways are in full view of the Lord, and he examines all his paths. The evil deeds of a wicked man ensnare him; the cords of his sin hold him fast. He will die for lack of discipline, led astray by his own great folly.

Proverbs 5: 1–23 NIV

The Days of Heaven on Earth Can be Yours

Form your own future with the words you speak. If things are not right within you, they will never be right around you. You also create your kids' future by what you speak into their lives. Love wisdom like a sweetheart; make wisdom a beloved member of your family.

You should get real about you. However, do not be too hard on yourself. Know that people are able to go to school to learn about everything except marriage and relationships, and few really teach on how to love and honor your spouse and family because this is something that is usually learned at home when growing up (if you were paying attention). You can also learn this when you are open and honest with yourself about what you need to learn about having a better marriage.

In coming into marriage, the two people should be whole: unique, with established standards, integrity and excellence not needy and in emotional, spiritual, physical, financial or moral disarray, hoping for a mate to complete them and provide all that is lacking. Marriage will show you who you truly are, because it will test your very last nerve. But it helps when you can celebrate your mate's uniqueness so that you can get from where you are to where you need to be. Marital bliss can be achieved; all you have to do is make a decision to make it so. It doesn't get any better than to live the rest of your life with someone who loves you and is committed to you in every way possible, someone who has your best interest at heart. Make it pleasurable, so that you and your mate can live the days of Heaven on Earth… as you Forever Please and Excite each other!

Benilda Nya

Part Three

Monthly Holidays and Event Coaching

January

Flower: Carnation, Snowdrop

Birthstone: Garnet–*constancy*

New Year's Day
Celebrated first in ancient Babylon about 4000 years ago, New Year's Day is the most ancient and universal of all holidays, and it often differs according to one's culture.

New Year's Day Traditions
New Year's Day is a day of parades, sporting events and new years resolutions. The Tournament of Roses Parade dates back to 1886, and it is followed by the Rose Bowl college football game.

To bring good luck
On the first day of the new year, eating anything in the shape of a circle is thought to bring good fortune by many cultures, because it represents "coming full circle." In most parts of the United States it is believed that eating legumes including black-eyed peas, as well as eating pig or cabbage is a sign of the expected prosperity for the new year.

For good luck, some cultures also believe in eating twelve grapes within the first few minutes of the new year, one for every month. In Israel, they eat apples dipped in honey on New Year's Day to bring a sweet year. The French, cheer the New Year with wine, champagne and a really special New Year's cake as a symbol of the sweet New Year that everyone wishes.

Another symbol that is connected with the New Year's celebration is that of a baby. This dates as far back as ancient Greece and Egypt as a universal symbol of rebirth, and it still finds its way into our modern celebrations as it represents the "baby New Year," in which all good things are possible.

"Auld Lang Syne"
Since the 1700s, the song, "Auld Lang Syne," is sung at the stroke of midnight in almost every English-speaking country in the world to bring in the new year. An old Scotch tune, "Auld Lang Syne" literally means "old long ago," "days gone by," "long long ago," or simply, "the good old days."

Meaningful Traditions and Things To Do On New Year's Day

New Year's Resolutions
The good old new years resolution tradition is said to have started with the Babylonians. Since so many of us make New Year's resolutions for a positive change, this is one of the most positive holidays that we can celebrate.

With this New Year comes the opportunity for a fresh and new start, as we say goodbye to the old year.

-Celebrating Tips
1. *New Year's Resolutions: Buy two 8X10 notebooks, one for each of you. Take time out with your spouse (include your children if they are old enough), talk about the things that you would like to accomplish for the new year as a couple as a family, and as individuals. Write down your personal and business goals, your "Mission" and "Vision" statements. Make your "Vision" board by cutting out pictures from magazines and newspapers with the things (clothes, car, home, toys) and situations/life style (your business, desired salary, net-worth, giving to your favorite foundation, etc.) that you want. Create a definite plan for carrying out your goals. Commit to reading your goals, mission and vision statements with passion twice daily. Once in the morning, soon after waking up and in the evening before going to sleep. Look at your vision board daily and be motivated, optimistic and grateful. Choose a quiet corner or area in your house, provide comfortable sitting and use it only to go over your mission and vision statements as well as to go over your affirmations.*

2. *Make a tradition out of releasing balloon wishes. Buy helium balloons in the colors that symbolize your desires for the new year. Purple means - power, royalty, luxury or elegance. Red - love, courage, desire, strength, determination, excitement or passion. Yellow - happiness, comfort, attention-grabbing, intellectual energy or optimism. Orange - stimulation, creativity, health or*

change. Green - well-being, nature, calm, growth, harmony or relaxation. Blue - peace, loyalty, honor, professionalism or trust. Gold - prosperity, wealth or wisdom. Silver - rich or glamour. Pink - sweet, playful or romance. Write each of your desires on paper, then attach each wish to the corresponding color balloon with a ribbon and release them into the sky within the first few minutes of the new year, say your affirmations for each goal and desire as they fly away. (Make a copy of the goals & desires you sent off and declare your affirmations daily and work your plan for achieving them.)

3. You can visit your family, friends and neighbors. Bring them some treats like cakes or cookies and your best wishes for the New Year.

4. Another great way to start the New Year is by helping those in need and by giving the gift of hope to those in need of motivation.

5. Include your children if they are old enough to participate. Please take pictures!

6. End the first day of the year at home by… Making an excellent dinner with all the trimmings, and please use your finest dinner wear.

Tu B'Shevat – Observed in January or February

Jewish Holidays happen on a different day every year because, the Jewish calendar coordinates with the rotation of the earth about its axis (a day), the revolution of the moon about the earth (a month), and the revolution of the earth about the sun (a year).

OTHER OBSERVANCES FOR THIS MONTH

- **National Blood Donor Month** – If possible, donate blood and encourage others to do so.
- **National Thank You Month** – Say thank you more often.
- **National Eye Care Month** – Visit your eye care physician and have your eyes and those you love checked.
- **National Book Month** – Start a book club.
- **Epiphany**
- **Save the Eagles Day**

- **Amelia Earheart Day**

- **Ben Franklin's Birthday**

- **Martin Luther King Jr. Day**

- **Christa McAuliffe**

- **Chinese New Year**

- Celebrating Tips

Celebrate the Chinese New Year. Join an oriental friend in their celebration or have a Chinese New Year dinner party (with some of the traditional foods), dress up in traditional Chinese clothing, decorate the house, play Chinese music and end with some fire works outside the house and in the" bedroom."

Super Bowl Sunday
-Celebrating Tips

Find out what he would like to do for Super Bowl Sunday. Have a super bowl party, for him and his friends. Find out if other wives are willing to participate. Whether the party is in your home or someone else's, make all the preparations with the help of the other wives. In case the party is just for the guys in your house, go ahead and set up everything they will need and make sure the children won't interrupt (if you have any). If he is staying home to watch by himself, get his favorite snack foods, beverages, get a hat or T-shirt of the team he likes (and for you too, because you should join him). Even if you do not like football, this is one of those times when you should support his excitement.

February

Flower: Violet, Primrose, Begonia

Birthstone: Amethyst–*sincerity*

Make this, a Valentine's Month, not just Day

-Celebrating Tips
1. *Give him a Valentine's gift every day for the month of February.*
2. *Very special sexual pleasure can also be part of this: dress up as a naughty nurse, a sexy cowgirl, etc. Wear different hair color wigs in several styles.*
3. *Play with different themes: Cleopatra, sexy dancer, sexy pinup girl posing for pictures, etc.*

Black History Month
Black History Month is a celebration to remember and learn more about the history and culture of black Americans.

National Freedom Day
Commemorates the signing of the 13th Amendment outlawing slavery on February 1, 1865 by President Lincoln.

Mardi Gras/Fat Tuesday
Celebrated on the day before Ash Wednesday. It occurs anytime between February 3rd and March 9th depending on when Easter is held that year.
"Let the Good Times Roll!"
-Celebrating Tips
1. *Plan a trip to New Orleans for Mardi Gras.*
2. *Have a Mardi Gras style dinner party: music, food, beads, etc. (Plan it together with him.)*

Religious Holidays
-Celebrating Tips

1. *Celebrate your maker! A family that prays together and puts God first has a better chance of survival and happiness, so praise your spouse for their spiritual strength and/or leadership.*

2. *Statistics show that couples that do not pray together have a higher divorce rate than those that pray together.*

Valentine's Day

February 14th is the traditional day to express your love for each other. Celebrate this spirit of love by sending a valentine, giving candy or other gifts.

There are two different legends of why we celebrate Valentine's Day... One legend started in Rome, when the Emperor, Claudius II, was involved in many bloody and unpopular campaigns. "Claudius the Cruel" as he was called, was having a difficult time getting soldiers to join his military leagues. He believed that the reason was that Roman men did not want to leave their loved ones. So, he cancelled all marriages and engagements in Rome.

The good Saint Valentine, who was a priest in Rome, in the year 269 A.D., together with his friend Saint Marius, defied Claudius and continued to perform marriages in secret. When Valentine's actions were discovered, he was sentenced to be beaten to death and have his head cut off.

While in prison, it is believed that Valentine fell in love with a young girl, who may have been his jailor's daughter, who visited him during his confinement. Before his death on the14th day of February, it is alleged that he wrote her a letter, which he signed "From Your Valentine"

In 496 A.D., Pope Gelasius set aside February 14 to honor St. Valentine.

Happy Valentine's Day, Darling

- *Start by having a "Valentine" theme dinner the night before Valentine's Day.* PINK and RED balloons, heart shaped dessert, table cloth, chair covers, napkins, wine glasses, water goblets, candles, pink champagne/ rose wine or pink beverage. Put some red in the food, too: red cabbage, onions, tomatoes or peppers. Choose red meat or pink salmon. Wear a pink or red outfit (which is his favorite color on you?). Have a red shirt for him to change into. If you have children old enough to enjoy the "Valentine" celebration dinner, let them help you put it together and have something red or pink for them to wear, also. (Have your kid(s) make or buy a valentine card for Dad & Mom.) Do not forget the music. If possible, you could hire a harpist to play during dinner.

- *On Valentine morning, kiss him & say: "Happy Valentine's Day, Darling/Baby/Pet name."* Give him his Valentine's card and gift. This gift could be something you know he wanted: tickets to a concert or sporting event, some sporting equipment, an accessory for his car/truck or something to match or add to an existing piece of clothing or jewelry. If you buy him more than one gift (shirt, pants, shoes, etc.), spread the giving throughout the day. In case he is a hunting or fishing enthusiast, you could also consider giving him a weekend trip where he can participate in these activities.

- *Whether you are going out to dinner or having an intimate dinner at home on "Valentines Day," dress and look your best.* Dress and smell the way you know he likes. Use excellent table and social manners. If he looks handsome or sexy, tell him. Tell him what you love and admire about him (how he treats you, his patience with the kids, his tidiness, understanding, courage, hard work, his problem solving skills, the way he helps around the house). Throughout the evening: look at him, flirt with him, smile at him and caress him. Kiss him on his eyes, lips and cheeks. The conversation should be positive and Romantic.

Benilda Nya

End Valentine's Month by:

1. *Having a relaxing but sexy dinner with music and cheek-to-cheek dancing at home, with all the trimmings and etiquette. Plan it together with your spouse*

2. *Write him a sexy letter to thank him for... Whatever he did for you/with you on Valentine's Day, weekend, or month and have it delivered along with an arrangement of assorted color roses (you are everything to me), have it delivered to him at work or surprise him when he gets home. Sign the letter with your lips in his favorite color & spray it with his favorite perfume.*

OTHER OBSERVANCES FOR THIS MONTH:

- **American Heart Month** – Keep a healthy heart.

- **National Dental Month** – A healthy mouth = Better health.

- **Chocolate Lovers Month**

- **National Bird Feeding Month**

- **Tu B'Shevat** – January or February

- **Purim** – February or March

- **Groundhog Day**

- **Ash Wednesday** – It occurs anytime between February 6th and March 9th, depending on when Easter is held that year.

- **Boy Scout Day**

- **Presidents' Day**

March

-Celebrating Tips
Start his month right… Excite him with five minutes of "sexual joy" at midnight or as soon as he wakes up in the morning.

Read Across America Day/Dr. Suess Birthday
-Celebrating Tips
Read poems to each other.

Palm Sunday
This is held on the Sunday before Easter Sunday, anytime between March and April, depending on when Easter is held that year.

St. Patrick's Day
-Celebrating Tips
Have a St. Patrick's Day theme dinner; don't forget the music.

First Day of Spring
-Celebrating Tips
1. *After breakfast, play some music and start your Spring-cleaning. In the middle of cleaning stop and call him over to join you in one of the closets and give him a little "spring" cleaning and tell him that this is his reward for helping you (if he has been helping you).*
2. *Decorate your home with spring flowers.*

Pesach (Passover) – March or April

Good Friday
It occurs anytime between March and April, depending on when Easter is held that year.

Easter Sunday
It occurs anytime between March 22nd and April 25th, on the first Sunday after the first full moon after March 20th.

ADDITIONAL OBSERVANCES FOR THIS MONTH

- **Purim** – February or March

- **National Nutrition Month** – Eat healthy and smart, and exercise

- **National Women's History Month** – Discover women's forgotten multicultural history and heritage.

- **Save Your Vision Week** – 1st week in March

- **Ash Wednesday** – February or March depending on when Easter is held that year.

- **Girl Scout Week 10-16**

- **National Poison Prevention Week** – 3rd week in March

- **Sea Turtles nesting period begins in Florida**

- **Daylight Savings Time** – Set clocks forward 1 hour

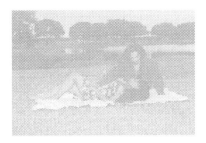

(Place a spring picture of the two of you here.)

April

Flower: Sweet Pea, Daisy, Freesia

Birthstone: Diamond–*innocence*

April Fools'/All Fool's Day
-Celebrating Tips

Play a nice trick on him, example: Babe, remember the shirt that you liked at_____, I was going to get you one, but I couldn't... TA DA, I got you TWO in different colors!

April 15th Taxes Due
-Celebrating Tips

Put on a business suit (stockings and sexy underwear) and pull your hair up, wear some reading glasses, act like an IRS agent and call him in (the home office or bedroom) for an "audit."

Earth Day
-Celebrating Tips

1. *Go to your favorite beach or park together and clean it up a bit.*
2. *Celebrate earth day; have dinner at home with him, "a la nude."*

Administrative Professionals Day / Week
-Celebrating Tips

Celebrate your good employees: give them their gifts and/or take them out to lunch, see if your husband can join you, or join him with his staff. (Definitely have your husband join you if you want to take your male staff out to eat.)

Arbor Day – Date varies from state to state from January to May
-Celebrating Tips

1. *Dedicate a forest, or a tree, in a park to your spouse or family.*
2. *To show your consideration and optimism for our planet, plant a tree with your mate and family.*

OTHER OBSERVANCES FOR THIS MONTH

- **Pesach / Passover** – March or April

- **Cancer Control Month**

- **Alcohol Awareness Month**

- **Patriots' Day**

- **Palm Sunday** – March or April

- **Good Friday** – March or April

- **Easter** – March or April

- **Patriot's Day**

- **Ascension Day** – This date varies by different faiths and religions.

May

Flower: Lily of the Valley, Lily

Birthstone: Emerald–*love, success*

Cinco de Mayo
-Celebrating Tips
1. *Celebrate Cinco de Mayo. Learn about the Mexican culture. Go to a Mexican restaurant for dinner.*
2. *Have a Mexican style dinner party with mariachi band and all.*

National Teachers Day / Teacher Appreciation Week – First Tuesday in May / First Full week in May
-Celebrating Tips
Great Teachers Make Great Schools… Don't forget the gifts for Teacher's Day; even a simple "thank you" card will be appreciated.

National Day of Prayer – 1st Thursday in May
-Celebrating Tips
1. *Pray with the spouse/kids for the country, its leaders and your friends, etc.*
2. *Join your church, synagogue or community in a prayer service or event.*

Mother's Day – 2nd Sunday in May
-Celebrating Tips
If you are a Mom, know that your kids are a gift from God; they are like a blank tape, recording from day one what they see you and your husband say and do.

Nurses Day – May 12th
-Celebrating Tips
Don't forget the gifts for your favorite nurses and celebrate the good nurses in your local Hospital. You and your mate should treat them to lunch/dinner and gifts.

Police Week – Week in which May 15 occurs
-Celebrating Tips
Support your local police department.

Armed Forces Day – 3rd Saturday in May **"America Supports You"**
-Celebrating Tips
See how you can be a blessing to those who protect this Country.

Memorial Day – Last Monday in May
-Celebrating Tips
1. *Talk about what to do for Memorial Day weekend.*
2. Have a happy Memorial Day weekend!
National Safe Boating Week
-Celebrating Tips
If you own a boat, take the family boating. Or go to a lake in the park and play with a motorized toy boat, or go canoeing or paddle boat riding. You can also go boat window-shopping and pick out a boat that the family would love to own in the future.

ADDITIONAL OBSERVANCES FOR THIS MONTH

- **Lag B'Omer** – May

- **Shavu'ot** – May or June

- **Asian/Pacific American Heritage Month**

- **National Physical Fitness & Sports Month**

- **Steelmark Month**

- **Law day** – May 1st

- **Loyalty Day** – May 1st (display U.S. flag)

- **May Day** – May 1st – the Real Labor Day

- **Join Hands Day** – 1st Saturday in May

- **Peace officers Memorial Day** – 15th day of May

- **National Maritime Day** – 22nd Day of May

- **National Defense Transportation Day** – 3rd Friday in May

- **Peace Officers Memorial Day** – 15th day of May

(If you haven't done it yet, this is the time that you can start a Christmas savings account.)

June

Flower: Rose

Birthstone: pearl, alexandrite, moonstone—*health*

*N*ational Rose Month

Roses date far back to pre-historic days. They are more than 33 million years old and have been used among friends and lovers to send all sorts of messages, and they are used for many reasons.

-Celebrating Tips

1. *On June 1st, send him 10 (yellow & orange) Roses. Let the card say: "Passionate thoughzts of you… my perfect 10."*
2. *End Rose Month by preparing a luxurious and romantic bubble bath for the both of you. Let a poster size note greet him at the door with instructions to follow the rose petal trail (frame the poster with roses). Let the rose petal trail lead to the bathroom where you have candlelight, music, finger food and some champagne, sprinkle the bubble bath with lots of rose petals. Caress and kiss him, have a flirtatious conversation as you wash and feed each other. Make yummy and passionate love to him.*

Famous Rose Quotes

-What's in a name? That which we call a rose/By any other name would smell as sweet. – William Shakespeare, Romeo and Juliet act II, sc. Ii
- O, my love's like a red, red rose/That's newly sprung in June. – Robert Burns, A Red, Red Rose
- Rose is a rose is a rose is a rose. – Gertrude Stein, Sacred Emily (1913), a poem well used in Geography and plays.

- Father's Day – 3rd Sunday in June
-Celebrating Tips

1. Involve your child/children in all the plans and activities to celebrate their dad.
2. Serve him breakfast in bed every weekend in June.
3. Surprise him with something really special every day or weekend in June.

4. If he is a good Dad: tell him that you are very proud of his Fatherly skills.

5. Have your child/children make or buy a father's day card for dad.

6. If your child/children have a talent, help them to put together a special performance for dad.

7. Give a party to honor him.

8. Rent his dream car for the week/weekend/day, for him to drive.

9. Rent his dreamboat or yacht and go with the family for a leisurely cruise.

10. Give him a weekend get away with the guys (you can get together with the wives of his friends and plan to give them a trip) hunting or fishing, (some tickets to the sports event of the year, or a concert with his favorite artist). A car/truck, tire rims or accessories for his car/truck. How about that lawnmower, sports equipment, or outfit he's been dreaming about?

ADDITIONAL OBSERVANCES FOR THIS MONTH

- **National Dairy Month**

- **Shavu'ot** – May or June, 50 days following Passover.

- **Ascension Day – Christian** – Observed in May or June

- **Atlantic Hurricane Season Begins** – June 1st

- **World Environment Day** – June 5th

-**Celebrating Tips**

Help your city organize a clean-up campaign, give a tree planting party or celebrate with a green concert and increase recycling awareness.

- **Philippines Independence Day** – June 11th

- **National Flag Week** – Week of June 14th – Display the flag of the United States.

- **Flag Day** – June 14th

- **Honor America Days** – June 14th thru July 4th

- **Juneteenth** – 19th day of June. Also called "Freedom Day" or "Emancipation Day." It's the oldest known holiday to commemorate the end of slavery: June 19,1865.

- **Emancipation Day** – Date Varies in the United States, Puerto Rico and the Caribbean.

- First Day of Summer – June 20th or 21st

Timed with the Summer Solstice.

-Celebrating Tips

1. *Celebrate the first day of summer with a picnic theme dinner, including the short pants.*
2. *Stay up all night on Solstice Eve and welcome the rising Sun at dawn.*

- St. Baptiste Day – 24th day of June – French-Canadian

- Ascension Day – Christian – Observed in May or June

- Helen Keller's Birthday – June 27th

- Paul Bunyan – June 28th

(Make plans for the 4th of July; take a long weekend or your vacation that week.)

July

Tisha B'Av – July or August

Canada Day – July 1st (July 2nd if July 1st is on a Sunday)

Independence Day – July 4th

-Celebrating Tips
1. *If you do not have any plans to go away for the July 4th weekend, take July 4th off and have a beach party, invite family and friends.*
2. *Go ahead, take July 4th off along with him and go for a picnic or spend the day at your favorite hotel and enjoy the fire works at night. Give him your own version of fireworks!*

Bastille Day – 14th day of July – French National Holiday

Parents' Day – 4th Sunday in July

-Celebrating Tips
1. *Invite the parents over for a cookout to celebrate Parent's Day.*
2. *Give them an award for being the best parents (a plaque, medal or trophy).*

August

Flower: Gladiolus, Poppy

Birthstone: Jade, Peridot, Sardonyx – *married, happiness*

-Celebrating Tips
Buy him a pair of Jade, Peridot or Sardonyx cuff links or a ring to celebrate your happy marriage.

Tisha B'Av – July or August

Ramadan – 9th Month of the Muslim Calendar – August or September
Every year Islamic holidays happen earlier and they don't always occur in the same season.

Friendship Day – 1st Sunday in August
Honor your good friends and let them know that they are greatly valued.
-Celebrating Tips
1. Get together with your friends and have a brunch party, hand out gifts or medals to acknowledge their wonderful contribution to your life.
2. Be a good neighbor.

Assumption Day – 15th day of Aug – Christian

National Aviation Day – 19th day of August – Orville Wright's Birthday 1871
-Celebrating Tips
1. If he likes airplane's, then surprise him with a model airplane that he can put together, or give him a remote control toy airplane.
2. If he is a pilot who always wanted his own airplane, give him his own (real) airplane to fly.

Women's Equality Day – August 26th
-Celebrating Tips
Be proud of being a woman. Be beautiful inside and out. Keep expanding in wisdom.

Make plans for Labor Day.

September

-Celebrating Tips
Buy him a pair of Sapphire cuff links.

Labor Day – 1st Monday in September
-Celebrating Tips
1. *Go away for the weekend or spend it doing something you both enjoy.*
2. Have a happy Labor Day weekend!

Ramadan – 9th Month of the Muslim Calendar – August or September

Islamic Eid ul-Fitr

Rosh Hashanah (Feast of Trumpets) – September
Jewish Holidays happen on a different day every year, and they begin in the fall starting with the celebration of the High Holy Days of Rosh Hashanah and Yom Kippur. The Jewish calendar coordinates with the rotation of the earth about its axis (a day), the revolution of the moon about the earth (a month), and the revolution of the earth about the sun (a year). All of the Jewish Holidays start at sundown the night before.

Yom Kippur – September - October

Grandparents Day – 1st Sunday after Labor Day in September
Honor your grandparents. Talk to your children about the wealth of information and character development that their grandparents can give. Grandparents can also celebrate their grandchildren and show them love. Grandparents Day is a day to further strengthen the spirit of love and respect for our elders.

-Celebrating Tips

1. *Have a family get-together. Play old family music; sing those old songs with grandpa and/or grandma, dance the old dances. Ask grandma to share her cooking recipes.*
2. *Let the grandparents tell the stories of their life, and how it was for them growing up.*
3. *Show the children and/or Grandchildren the old photographs in your family albums.*
4. *Put together a family tree photo album.*
5. *Talk about your family's ethnic or religious beliefs.*

Patriot Day – September 11, 2001
-Celebrating Tips

Take time out today to pray for the families and survivors of 9/11/01. Pray also for world peace and for God's protection over the U.S.A. and the world from terrorists.

National Hispanic Heritage Month – Sept. 15th – Oct. 15
-Celebrating Tips

1. *Celebrate with your local Hispanic community.*
2. *Sign up for Salsa classes this month as a couple.*
3. *Go visit a Spanish museum or Art gallery.*
4. *Go out to dinner at a Latin restaurant. Make sure that you dress sexy. Be very flirtatious in the way you talk and caress him. Tell him in Spanish: "hay papi que rico te vez." Translation: "oh baby, you look delicious." Say it with passion. (For more "foreign love talk" see Part Seven, page 216.)*

Stepfamily Day – 16th day of September
-Celebrating Tips

If you are a stepfamily, go and do something fun and let each other know how much you love and appreciate each other.

Constitution Day & Week – September 17th

International Day Of Peace – 21st

Native American Day – 4th Friday in September
-Celebrating Tips

1. *Visit your local Native American museum or art gallery.*

2. Celebrate with your local Native Americans.
3. Learn about the Native Americans.
4. Surprise your spouse for dinner with a tipi in the living room or the backyard; dress up as "Pocahontas," serve dinner and eat as the Native Americans. Make love in your tipi (on some fury rugs) and sleep there, if possible.

First day of Autumn
-Celebrating Tips
Bake an apple or pumpkin pie.

Enjoy the Fall Season

*G*o on a hayride (hug and kiss)

....

*R*ent a cabin in the mountains for a long weekend

....

*T*ake a walk or a drive and enjoy the beautiful color changes

....

*I*f either of you enjoy the sport of hunting, go on a hunting trip

....

*M*ake out on a pile of fallen leaves, in a private
place at the park or in your backyard

Benilda Nya

169

October

Flower: Magnolia

Birthstone: Opal, Tourmaline–*hope*

National Hispanic Heritage Month Sept. 15th – Oct. 15th
-Celebrating Tips
1. Learn together about the Hispanic Heritage.
2. *CELEBRATE Hispanic month…go out dancing at a Latin club. Dress very feminine & sexy; flirt with him. Later, make your lovemaking "muy caliente" (very hot). (For more foreign " love talk," see Part Seven, page 212.)*

Yom Kippur – September – October

Sukkot – September – October

Shemi ni Atzeret – September – October

Simchat Torah – October

National Breast Cancer Month

National Disability Employment Awareness Month

Child Health Day – 1st Monday
-Celebrating Tips
Help your child to understand the benefits of taking care of their health.

National Children's Day – 8th
-Celebrating Tips
Show the children in your life how much you love and value them.

Leif Erikson Day – 9th

National School Lunch Week (9-13)
-Celebrating Tips
Call your kids' school, and see if there is anything you can do for "Lunch Week."

Columbus Day Observed – 2nd Monday
Display U.S. flag

Thanksgiving – Canada – 2nd Monday

White Cane Safety Day – 15th

National Forest Products Week (15-21)
-Celebrating Tips
If you have kids old enough, get with your mate & ask them to do a research on forest products.

National Boss Day – 16th
-Celebrating Tips
1. *Why don't you and your husband take your boss (yours and/or his) and his/her significant other out to lunch or dinner?*
2. *Give your boss a gift.*
3. *Give a breakfast to honor your boss.*

Boss's Day

If you are "The Boss," make sure that you are a great boss. According to their expertise, pay them well. Be fair; encourage, praise and reward your employees (for a job well-done, an employee can get a spa day or financial bonus). Be concerned with their overall needs, and have a support system so that they will know your company is worth their loyalty, dedication and hard work.

Give your business or office a "happy" makeover. Find out what can make your employees happy at work, so that the business and production can increase. HAPPINESS = less stress, less sick time taken, better creativity, improved interactions with co-workers and clients, promotions and increased success and more profits.

If possible, provide day care (for a small fee) on the premises. You can also help your employees release stress: make available a room with plants, a water fountain, floor mats, CD player with relaxing music, a TV-video player where they can play yoga, tai chi or Qigong videos to de-stress. A place where they can do deep breathing and stretching exercises for about fifteen minutes a day (it could be before the start of the day or some time in the middle of the workday). Don't allow eating lunch at the desk while working (that goes for the boss, also).

The lunch/break room should be nicely decorated (plants, water fountain) and well stocked. (Your employees should feel well cared for if you want them to perform great for you. At the same time, they need to know that you mean business and you need to run your company at its best.)

PLEASE, let your employees enjoy their day off and vacations, do not call them for anything. Also, do not micro-manage your people. If you need to, get rid of incompetent or lazy employees. Hire the right people even if it takes time to do so.

If you are the "employee," make sure that you are trustworthy, responsible and dedicated. Constantly increase the knowledge that concerns your duties and your professional goals. Skilled happy employees get promoted or asked to become a partner in the company.

Benilda Nya

- A wise man's heart guides his mouth, and his lips promote instruction. Proverbs 16: 23

Like the coolness of snow at harvest time is a trustworthy messenger (employee) to those who send him; he refreshes the spirit of his masters (employer). Proverbs 25: 13

Sweetest Day – 3rd Saturday
-Celebrating Tips
Give candy, flowers or gifts to the people in your life who are aged, sick, orphaned children, and the ones who are caring.

Mother-In-Law Day – 4th Sunday
-Celebrating Tips
Invite the in-laws (your parents and his) out to brunch or dinner, if possible.

United Nations day – 24th

Halloween
-Celebrating Tips

Not everybody likes to celebrate Halloween, but you can make it fun and wholesome for your kids by having your own party without the scary costumes.

Throw a Romantic Costume Ball

Get together with your mate and pick a romantic era or romantic couples throughout history and have a "couples" costume party based on the way they dressed. Invite your friends, family, neighbors, business partners and co-workers.

Benilda Nya

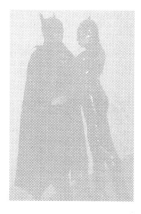

(Place a picture of both of you in a costume here.)

November

Flower: Chrysanthemum, Orchid

Birthstone: Topaz–*fidelity*

National American Indian Heritage Month

Good Nutrition Month

Aviation Month

Daylight-Saving Time Ends (set clocks back)

All Saints' Day – 1st

All Souls' Day – 2nd

Guy Fawkes Day – 5th - United Kingdom

Veteran's Day – 11th U.S. End WW1

Remembrance Day – 11th - Canada - End WW1 - 1918

Armistice Day – 11th - Europe - End WW1 - 1918

Thanksgiving Day – 3rd Thursday
-Celebrating Tips
Smile, be happy, and use your table etiquette; be a good hostess.

Give Thanks

- ❤ Thanksgiving Day is what it is, "Thanksgiving." Make it a family affair by having your older kids prepare and read the story of the Pilgrims and the Indians. They could even wear costumes and make a little play out of it. If you do not have any kids but are having young nieces and nephews come over, have them read the "Thanksgiving" story.

- ❤ If the dinner is in your home, the thanksgiving prayer should go around the table starting at your husbands left, as each person gives thanks for whom and for what they are thankful. It should end with you or your husband.

174

❤ **T**he carving of the turkey should be done by either you or your husband (who ever does it best), unless the grandfather has been the one to do it throughout the years, or any other person that you agree does a great job at carving the turkey.

Benilda Nya

Gobble Gobble

❤ **S**ome men take great pride in cooking the turkey (and do a great job at it); so if your husband is one of them, let him have his fun. If he would also like to help with any other cooking, baking and cleaning, that is great especially, if you and your husband are the ones having the families over to your house for the dinner.

❤ **F**ind a homeless shelter to help: whether you donate food or your time by stepping out earlier in the day to help serve. Share your blessings; feed the hungry.

❤ **I**f he cannot miss his favorite team playing football, please talk it over with him and find the perfect time to serve dinner, so that your family can have his undivided attention. But please, no arguments or disagreements to spoil a happy time.

Benilda Nya

Take Joy in the Holidays

According to your religious and/or family traditions, make sure that you are a vital part of all the festivities. Make it one of the happiest and fun times in your home. This will also be a good example and support for your children (if you have any).

Benilda Nya

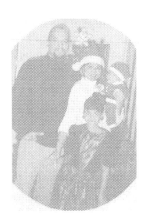

(Place a holiday family picture here.)

December

Flower: Hibiscus, Holly, Poinsettia

Birthstone: Turquoise, Zircon - *prosperity*

-Celebrating Tips
Build a snowman together.

-Celebrating Tips
1. *Buy yourself a sexy "Mrs. Santa" loungewear outfit to wear on Christmas Eve or Day.*
2. *Team work: wrap the Christmas gifts together, drink some eggnog, listen to Christmas songs, laugh, be happy.*

Ashura – December or January - This Islamic holiday is observed on the 10th of Muharram, the first month of the Islamic year.

Hanukkah – December, every few years in November

AIDS Awareness Day – 1st
-Celebrating Tips
Talk to your older children about the danger of HIV and AIDS.

Nat'l Pearl Harbor Remembrance Day – 7th

Human Rights Day – 10th

Wright Brother's Day – 17th
-Celebrating Tips
Play Captain and Co-pilot.

Pan American Aviation Day – 17th
-Celebrating Tips
Play Passenger and Flight Attendant.

Forefathers' Day – 21st

First Day of Winter – 21st or 22nd - The shortest day of the year
-Celebrating Tips
Go shopping for matching winter outfits.

National Regifting Day – Thursday before Christmas

Christmas Eve – 24th
-Celebrating Tips
Be a "good" Mrs. Santa.

Merry Christmas!

Gather up those Christmas lists and start the shopping. Time to withdraw from that Christmas account and start shopping.

....

If you have kids (and they can enjoy helping you choose the gifts), take them with you and your husband to do the shopping for your family, friends, Pastor/Rabbi/Minister/Priest, boss and co-workers.

....

Have a budget and stick to it. Instead of buying a gift for each person in a family, you can buy one thing that everybody can enjoy.

....

If your wife's or kids' list is longer than your budget, ask them to prioritize (1-5, five being the least desirable). But do not give away the element of surprise.

....

For Christmas you can give him a gift a day for the twelve Days of Christmas. Or for Hanukkah: give him one for each of the eight days.

....

Help each other to wrap the gifts, and play Christmas songs and drink some eggnog.

Benilda Nya

Join in the Reindeer games

Play Christmas music while having dinner.

. . . .

Go for a drive or walk to see the decorated homes and streets.

. . . .

If you have children or teens that are a part of their school, church or community Christmas play, make sure that you go with your husband to see them perform.

. . . .

Enjoy some of those Christmas plays and movies with your spouse and/or the whole family.

. . . .

Take your spouse and family to a Christmas amusement park; get on the rides with him/them; act silly, laugh, eat and have some fun.

. . . .

Get together with your friends, neighbors and/ or family, and give a fun Christmas party.

Benilda Nya

Oh, Christmas Tree

Shop for the Christmas tree together or
compliment him if he surprises you with it.

....

If he wants to help with the decorating of the tree let him have his fun.

....

If his thing is decorating the outside of the house, encourage him
with your praises, assist if he needs you and bring him some snacks.

....

Don't forget to hang the mistletoe, and kiss under it.

Benilda Nya

Exciting Him During the Holidays

If you have not yet told him how handsome he looks,
thanked him for his help with the decorating, or told
him how much you appreciate him helping you to pick
out the gifts; this will be a good time to do so!

....

Make your house beautiful and inviting. Always have something
ready to drink and to eat. Fresh-baked cookies or cake are always
nice. You could also have easy- to-prepare food on hand that
you can put together quickly for those unexpected guests.

....

If you have kids old enough to appreciate a compliment, make
sure that you thank them for their good behavior. If they helped
to decorate and keep the house clean, thank them for helping,
and if they are wearing something that looks great; tell them.

Benilda Nya

Christmas Day – 25th
Merry Christmas!
<u>**-Celebrating Tips**</u>
Be a good example of the Christmas spirit; be joyful and thankful in everything.

Kwanzaa – December 26th thru Jan. 1st

New Year's Eve – 31st

Have a Happy and Prosperous New Year, full of Romance!

Part Four

Flowers and Their Meaning

The Meaning Of Color For Flowers

When you give flowers or buy flowers for yourself, you can choose the mood and ambiance you want to create as well as the meaning and message you want to send. Yes, by simply choosing the kind of flower and the color(s) you can produce the environment you want to establish for yourself and others.

With the information about flowers in this section, you can be as creative and purposeful as you would like to be. When sending flowers to some one, add in the meaning on the card or letter so that they can be inspired and appreciate the flowers even more.

Purposeful Color

VIOLET – analogous with royalty, aristocracy, a symbol of faith and spirituality; it's energizing. Tell the recipient that they are extraordinary

BLUE – can improve your enthusiasm, it helps to heighten creativity, its soothing and it invites in a peaceful environment. Blue flowers impart a calm solution to our overly stressed lives and schedules

RED – represents love, vitality, passion & desire

ORANGE – the color of friendship, represents progress and sincerity, increase

YELLOW – admiration, gratefulness, provision, wisdom, lucidity, loyalty

INDIGO – perfect for people who multi-task/very busy people. Get in touch with deep feelings and show them. Helps to take it down a notch, increase on quality time

The Meaning Of Color For Roses

- ❤ **Red Roses:** "I love you." Passionate love. Romantic love. Admiration. Valor.
- ❤ **White Roses:** Innocence. Secrecy and silence. "I am worthy of you." Purity. Charm. Reverence. Humility. Spiritual love. "You are heavenly." Youthfulness.
- ❤ **Bridal White:** Happy love.
- ❤ **Yellow:** Joy. Gladness. Friendship. Devotion. Try to care. Welcome back. Remember me. Infidelity and jealousy.
- ❤ **Coral Roses:** Enthusiasm. Desire.
- ❤ **Orange:** Fascination. You are my secret love.
- ❤ **Light Peach:** Modesty of friendship.
- ❤ **Light Pink:** Grace. Gentility. Admiration. Sympathy.
- ❤ **Dark pink:** Say "Thank you." Appreciation. Gratitude.
- ❤ **Pink:** Perfect happiness. Love. "Thank you." Grace. Admiration.
- ❤ **Deep Burgundy:** "Unconscious beauty." Mourning.
- ❤ **Pale colored Roses:** Signify friendship.
- ❤ **Lavender:** Mean love at first sight.
- ❤ **Champagne:** You are tender and loving.
- ❤ **Red and White Together:** signify unity.
- ❤ **White and Purple Together:** Symbolic representations of purity and passion.
- ❤ **Pink and White:** I love you still and always will.
- ❤ **Yellow and Orange Together:** Passionate thoughts.
- ❤ **Red and Yellow Together:** Are an expression of congratulations or happy feelings.
- ❤ **Rose (tea):** I'll always remember you.
- ❤ **Rose (Christmas):** Peace and tranquility.
- ❤ **Rose (musk cluster):** Capricious beauty.
- ❤ **Rose (hibiscus):** Delicate beauty.
- ❤ **Black Rose:** You are my obsession. Death.
- ❤ **Assorted Color Roses Together:** You're everything to me.
- ❤ **A Crown made of Roses:** Signifies reward of merit or virtue.

When giving the flowers, use the meaning of it as part of the poem, love letter or note; you can also give the flowers along with a gift.

The Story of Roses

- ❤ **Thornless Rose:** Love at first sight.
- ❤ **Long Stemmed Rose:** "I will remember you always."
- ❤ **Short Stemmed Rose:** Sweetheart. Girlhood.
- ❤ **Rosebud:** Beauty and youth. A heart innocent of love.
- ❤ **Rosebud (white):** Girlhood; too young to love.
- ❤ **Rosebud (red):** Pure and lovely.
- ❤ **Rosebud (moss):** Confessions of love.
- ❤ **A Single Rose:** Any color – "I appreciate you."
- ❤ **A Single Rose:** Red in full bloom – "My love for you is unchanged," or "I still love you."
- ❤ **2 Roses:** Taped or wired together to form a single stem signal an engagement or coming marriage.
- ❤ **2 Roses:** We both feel the same deep love. We share the same feelings.
- ❤ **3 Roses:** "I love you."
- ❤ **A full blown Rose placed over two buds:** Secrecy.
- ❤ **6 Roses:** "I want to be yours."
- ❤ **7 Roses:** "I'm head over heels in love with you."
- ❤ **9 Roses:** "We'll be together for ever." Eternal love.
- ❤ **10 Roses:** "You are perfect."
- ❤ **11 Roses:** "You are the one I cherish." "You are my treasured one."
- ❤ **12 Roses:** "I want you to be mine!" Pleasurable combination. Combined likeness.
- ❤ **13 Roses:** "We are for ever friends." Secret admirer.
- ❤ **15 Roses:** "I apologize." "I'm truly sorry."
- ❤ **20 Roses:** "My feelings towards you are sincere."
- ❤ **21 Roses:** "I'm totally committed to you." "I'm dedicated to you."
- ❤ **24 Roses:** Keep me lovingly in your mind, all the time. "I cannot get you out of my mind." "Forever yours."
- ❤ **25 Roses:** "Well done." "Bravo." "Congratulations."
- ❤ **33 Roses:** "My love for you is INTENSE." Affection.
- ❤ **36 Roses:** "Reminiscing our romantic time together." I am experiencing romantic affections towards you every time you come near me.
- ❤ **40 Roses:** "My love for you is genuine."
- ❤ **44 Roses:** My vow to you is faithful and consistent. Unchangeable pledge.

- ♥ **50 Roses:** This is "Regretless/Unconditional Love."
- ♥ **56 Roses:** My darling.
- ♥ **66 Roses:** Successful love affair.
- ♥ **99 Roses:** "I will love you all the days of my life." Love with understanding makes love eternal.
- ♥ **100 Roses:** The most pleasurable marriage of the century. We are dedicated to each other forever.
- ♥ **101 Roses:** "There is no one else for me but you." Totally committed to you.
- ♥ **108 Roses:** "Will you marry me." "Will you take my hand in holy matrimony?"
- ♥ **111 Roses:** Endless love.
- ♥ **123 Roses:** Free love.
- ♥ **144 Roses:** I love you day and night, forever.
- ♥ **365 Roses:** Thinking of you every day. I love you each and every day.
- ♥ **999 Roses:** "I will love you 'till the end of time."
- ♥ **1001 Roses:** Faithful love. 'Till forever.
- ♥ **Rose leaves:** Long for. Hope.

More Flowers

A

Amaranth	Immortal Love
Amaryllis	Beauty; Dramatic; Pride
Anthurium	Hospitality
Aster	Elegance; Variety; Symbol of Love; Daintiness, Contentment
Azalea	Temperance; First love; Romance; Fragile Passion; Love

B

Baby's Breath	Innocence
Bamboo	Steadfastness; Strength; Loyalty
Begonia	Beware; Fanciful Nature; Be Cordial; Deep thoughts
Bird of Paradise	Magnificence; Freedom; Good Perspective; Given at ninth wedding anniversary

C

Cactus	Endurance; Warmth
Carnation, General	Fascination; Woman; Divine Love
Carnation, Pink	I'll Never Forget You; Motherly Love; Gratitude
Carnation, Red	My Heart Aches For You; Admiration; I Hold You in High Esteem; Respect; Deep Love, Friendship
Carnation, Purple	Capriciousness
Carnation, Solid Color	Yes
Carnation, Striped	No; Refusal; Sorry, I Can't Be With You; Wish I Could Be With You
Carnation, White	Sweet and Lovely; Innocence; Pure Love; Woman's Good Luck Gift
Carnation, Yellow	You Have Disappointed Me; Rejection; The 13th wedding anniversary flower
Chrysanthemum	(in general) Cheerfulness; Optimism; Rest; Truth; Long Life; joy; You are a Wonderful Friend

Chrysanthemum, Red	I Love you
Chrysanthemum, White	Loyal love, Truthfulness
Chrysanthemum, Yellow	Slighted Love; Secret Admirer; Chivalry
Cyclamen	Resignation; Good-bye

D

Daffodil	Chivalry; Rebirth; New beginnings; Regard; Unrequited Love; You're the Only One; Given for the 10th wedding anniversary
Daisy	Love that conquers all; Innocence; Loyal Love; I'll keep your secret; Purity; Gentleness; Given for the fifth wedding anniversary
Daisy, Red	Joy
Daisy, White	Innocence; Truth
Daisy, Yellow	I will try hard to earn your Love
Gerbera Daisy	Cheerfulness
Dandelion	Faithfulness; Happiness; Wishes come True; Oracle of Time and Love

E

Eucalyptus	Protection

F

Fern	Sincerity; Magic; Fascination; Confidence; Shelter
Fern, Maidenhair	Secret bond of love
Freesia	Innocence; Thoughtfulness; Spirited
Fir	Time
Forget-Me-Not	True Love; Memories; Remember me forever
Forsythia	Anticipation
Fuschia	Amiability; Taste; Given for third wedding anniversary

G

Gardenia	Joy; My Secret Love; You are lovely

Gladiolus	Strength of Character; I am really Sincere; Flower of the gladiators
Gloxinia	Love at First Sight

H

Heather, Pink	"Good Luck"
Heather, Purple	Admiration; Beauty and Solitude
Heather, White	Protection; Wishes Will Come True
Hibiscus	Delicate Beauty
Holly	Domestic Happiness
Hyacinth, General	Games and Sports; dedicated to Apollo
Hyacinth, Blue	Constancy; Predictability; Reliable
Hyacinth, Purple	I am Sorry; Please Forgive me; Sorrow
Hyacinth, Red or Pink	Play
Hyacinth, White	Loveliness; I Will Pray for You
Hyacinth, Yellow	Jealousy
Hydrangea	Thank You for Understanding; Heartlessness

I

Iris	Faith; Wisdom; Valor; Your Friendship means so much to me; My Compliments; Fleur-de-lis; Emblem of France; Passion; Inspiration; Given for 25th wedding anniversary
Iris White	Purity
Iris Blue	Faith; Hope
Iris Yellow	Passion
Iris Purple	Wisdom; Compliments
Ivy	Fidelity; Friendship; Wedded Love; Affection; Marriage

J

Jasmine	Amiability; attracts wealth; Grace & Elegance
Jasmine, Red	Folly; Glee
Jasmine, Yellow	Timidity; Modesty

Jasmine Spanish	Sensuality
Jonquil	Love Me; Affection Returned; Violent Desire/ Sympathy

L

Larkspur	Open heart; Beautiful spirit
Larkspur, Pink	Fickleness
Larkspur, Purple	First love; Sweet Disposition
Larkspur, White	Joyful; Happy-go Lucky
Lavender	Success; Luck; Happiness; Constancy; Distrust
Lilac	Youthful; Confidence; Humility
Lilac, Mauve	"Do you still Love me?"
Lilac, Pink	Youth; Acceptance
Lilac, Purple	You are my first Love
Lilac, White	"My first Dream of Love"
Lily	Majesty; Wealth; Pride; Innocence; Purity
Lily, Calla	Majestic Beauty; I am in Heaven When I'm With You; Associated with the sixth wedding anniversary
Lily, Casablanca	Celebration
Lily, Day	Coquetry; Chinese Emblem for Mother
Lily, Orange	Flame; I burn for you; Hatred; Disdain
Lily, Pink	Youth and Acceptance; Romantic
Lily, Stargazer	I See Heaven in Your Eyes
Lily, Tiger	Wealth; Pride
Lily, White	Majesty; Purity; Virginity; It's heavenly to be with you; My love is pure and innocent
Lily, Yellow	Live for the Moment; I'm Walking on Air
Lily- Of -The- Valley	Humility; Sweetness; Return to Happiness; Tears of the Virgin Mary; You've Made My Life Complete
Lotus	Mystery and Truth

M

Magnolia	Dignity; Nobility; Splendid Beauty
Marigold	Desire for riches; Sacred Affection; Cruelty; Grief; Jealousy

Mistletoe	Kiss me; Affection; To Surmount Difficulties; Sacred Plant of India
Myrtle	Love; Mirth; Joy; Hebrew Emblem of Marriage
Myrrh	Gladness

N

Narcissus	Egotism; Formality; Stay as Sweet as You Are

O

Orchid	Love; Rare Beauty; Beautiful lady; Refinement; Magnificence; Chinese symbol for many children; Given at the 28th wedding anniversary; long life

P

Palm leaves	Victory and Success
Pansy	Thoughtful Recollection of you, Loyalty; Symbolic of the Trinity because of their three colors; Can be given at the first wedding anniversary
Poinsettia	"Be of Good Cheer"
Poppy, General	Imagination; Dreaminess; Eternal Sleep; Ninth wedding anniversary
Poppy, Oriental	Silence is Golden
Poppy, Red	Pleasure; Consolation
Poppy, Scarlet	Extravagance
Poppy, White	Consolation; Tranquility
Poppy, Yellow	Wealth; Success
Primrose	Satisfaction; Happiness; Young Love; I cannot live with out You

S

Snowdrop	Hope
Sunflower	Homage and Devotion
Sweet Pea	Departure; Blissful Pleasure; Lasting Pleasure; Thank You for a Lovely Time; Shyness

T

Tulip   Symbol of The Perfect Lover; Flower Emblem of
                             Holland
Tulip, Red   Believe Me; Declaration of Love
Tulip, Variegated   Beautiful Eyes
Tulip, Yellow   There's Sunshine in your Smile; I am hopelessly in
                             Love
Tulip, Cream   I will Love you forever

V

Violet   Modesty; Virtue; Demureness; Faithfulness; Given
                             for fiftieth wedding anniversary; Simplicity
Violet, Yellow   I Love My Country
Violet, Purple   Blue love; Thoughts of you
Violet, Blue   Watchfulness; Faithfulness; I'll always be true
Violet, White   Let's take a chance

W

Water Lily   Eloquence and Persuasion; Purity of Heart
Wisteria   Welcome

X

Xeranthemum   Cheerfulness under adverse conditions

Y

Yarrow   Health-giving; Sorrow

Z

Zinnia   Thinking of Friends not Present
Zinnia, Pink   Eternal Fondness
Zinnia, White   Goodness
Zinnia, Yellow   Daily Remembrance
Zinnia, Scarlet   Constancy

Part Five

More of His Favorite Things

His Favorite Romantic Songs

Name	Artist	Name	Artist

His Favorite Boogie Songs

Name	Artist	Name	Artist

*H*is Favorite Restaurants

Steakhouse-Asian-Sushi-Caribbean-Latin-Mexican-Italian-
Middle Eastern-European-Bar & Bistro-Seafood-Buffet-Barbeque-
Sandwiches & Subs-Soup & Salad-Café-Deli-Sports Café/
Bar-Pizza-Health Food-Fast Food-Breakfast-Lunch-Gourmet-
Bakery-Takeout-Ice Cream Shop-Smoothie-Vegetarian

Name/Type	*Location*	*Tel.*

*H*is Favorite Theatres

Movie-Playhouse-Performing Arts-Arena-Concert Hall-Stadium

Name/Type	*Location*	*Tel.*

His Favorite Supermarket & Pharmacy

Name/Type   Location   Tel.

_____

_____

_____

His Favorite Household Cleaning Brands

Laundry Detergent:_____

Fabric Softener:_____

Bleach:_____

Disinfectant:_____

Glass Cleaner:_____ **All Purpose Cleaner:**_____

Floor:_____

Bathroom:_____

Kitchen: Dishwashing:_____

Other:_____

His Favorite Food Brands

Type   Brand   Type   Brand

_____

_____

_____

_____

His Favorite Personal Hygiene Brands

Type   *Brand*

_____

_____

_____

His Favorite Bedding Brands

Thread Count:_____Bed Size:_____Mattress Type:_____

Circle His Favorite Styles: Traditional - Casual - Modern - Country - Romantic

Favorite Colors:_____

Circle His Favorites: Bed Spread - Comforter - Duvet Cover - Quilt - Blanket **Other:**_____

Pillow Size(s): Standard - King_____

Filling: Goose Down - Organic - Down Alternative_____

Decorative/Accent Pillows:_____

Fabrics: Cotton - Cotton Jersey - Egyptian Cotton - Flannel - Silky Satin Cotton Sateen - Organic **Other:**_____

Fabric Styles: Solid Colors - Stripes - Dots - Floral Prints - Lace - Pattern Animal Prints - Embroidered - Bordered

Designers:_____

Store Brands:_____

Organic Brands:_____

His Favorite Parks & Recreation

Name/Type   Location   Tel.

_____

_____

_____

His Favorite Area Attractions

Museums-Zoo-Library-Planetarium & Observatory-Seaquarium
Botanical Garden-Beach-Art Gallery

Name/Type   Location   Tel.

_____

_____

_____

His Favorite Airports

Name/Type   Location   Tel.

_____

_____

His Favorite Airlines

Name/Type   Location   Tel.

_____

_____

His Favorite Cruise Line

Name/Type   Location   Tel.

_____

_____

_____

His Favorite Electronic Brands

Name/Type   Location   Tel.

_____

_____

_____

_____

His Favorite Appliance Brands

Name/Type   Location   Tel.

_____

_____

_____

_____

Part Six

Birthdays, Anniversaries, Contacts and Notes

Birthdays and Anniversaries

Date	Name	Occasion

Special People & Contacts

Name:

Address:

Telephone: Email:

Name:

Address:

Telephone: Email:

Name:

Address:

Telephone: Email:

Name:

Address:

Telephone: Email:

Name:

Address:

Telephone: Email:

Name:

Address:

Telephone: Email:

Special People & Contacts

Name:

Address:

Telephone: **Email:**

Name:

Address:

Telephone: **Email:**

Name:

Address:

Telephone: **Email:**

Name:

Address:

Telephone: **Email:**

Name:

Address:

Telephone: **Email:**

Name:

Address:

Telephone: **Email:**

Special People & Contacts

Name:

Address:

Telephone: Email:

Name:

Address:

Telephone: Email:

Name:

Address:

Telephone: Email:

Name:

Address:

Telephone: Email:

Name:

Address:

Telephone: Email:

Name:

Address:

Telephone: Email:

Notes

Notes

Notes

Part Seven

Fanning the Flames of Romance

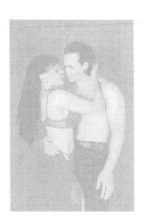

(Place a "sexy" picture here of the two of you.)

To fan the flames of romance…
Give each other sweet or sexy pet names

Boo

Bon Bon

Chocolate Delight

My Knight in Shining Armor

My Passion-tini (passion-martini)

Rico-Suave (Spanish: yummy & smooth)

Amore Mio (Italian: my love)

Mi Rey (Spanish: my king)

Ma Vie (French: my life)

My Banana Bliss

My Pleasure Toy

My Vanilla Joy

My Lollypop

My Sunshine

My Joy Stick

My Boy Toy

Sexy Hunk

Handsome

Eye Candy

Lover Boy

My Lover

Sweet or Sexy Expressions
In other languages

English	*French*	*Pronunciation*
- My Love =	Mon Amour	Mon Nah-Moor
- My Life =	Ma Vie	Mah Vee
- Kiss Me! =	Embrasse - Moil!	Ahn-Brah S Mwah
- Yes =	Oui	Wee
- Please =	Sil vous plait	Seel Voo Ple
- Thank you =	Merci	Mer-See
- Hello =	Bonjour	Bon Zhoor
- I'm sorry =	Je suis de sole	Zhuh Swee Da-Sola
- Good-bye =	Au Revoir	O Ruh-Vwahr
- Good morning =	Bonjour	Bon Zhoor
- Good night =	Bonne Nuit	Buhn Nwee
- With pleasure! =	Avec plaisir!	Ah-ve K Pla-Zeer
- Well Done! =	Bravo!	Brah-Vo

English	*Italian*	*Pronunciation*
- My Love =	Amore Mio	Ah-mo-re mee-o
- My Life =	Vita Mia	Vee-tah mee-ah
- Kiss Me! =	Baciami!	Bah-chah-mee
- Come Here! =	Venga qui	Ven-gah kwee
- With Pleasure! =	Con piacere!	Kon pee-ah-che-re

216

- Farewell My Love! = Addio Amore Mio!-------Ahd-dee-oh ah-moh-re mee-oh

- Perfect = Perfetto--------------------------------Pehr-feht-toh

- Hello & Good-bye = Ciao-------------------------------------Chah-oh

- Spicy = Piccante------------------------------Peek-kahn-teh

- Good = Buono--------------------------------Boo-oh-noh

English	Portuguese	Pronunciation
- Beautiful Woman =	Gata------------------------------------	Gah-tah
- Handsome Man =	Gato------------------------------------	Gah-toh
- Let's Get To It =	Vamos la-----------------------------	Vah-mooz lah

English	Spanish	Pronunciation
- Beautiful (F) =	Bella-----------------------------------	Bveh-yah
- Beautiful (M) =	Bello-----------------------------------	Bveh-yoh
- Yes =	Si---------------------------------------	See
- Hello =	Hola-----------------------------------	O-lah
- Good-bye =	Adios----------------------------------	Ah-dee-os
- Kiss Me! =	Besame!-------------------------------	Be-sah-me
- My Life =	Mi Vida-------------------------------	Mee vee-dah
- My Love =	Mi Amor------------------------------	Mee ah-mor
- Thank You =	Gracias--------------------------------	Grah-see-ahs

"*I Love You*"
In other languages

LANGUAGE	I LOVE YOU
1 - Arabic	Ana Behiback (to a male)
	Ana Behibek (to a female)
2 - Canadian	Sh'teme
3 - Chinese	Wo le Ni (Mandarin)
	Ngo oiy Ney a (Cantonese)
4 - Cherokee	Gvgeyuhi
5 - Czech	Miluji Te
6 - Danish	Jeg Elsker Dig
7 - Dutch	Ik Hou Van Jou
8 - Filipino	Mahal Kita
9 - French	Je T'aime, Je T'adore
10- German	Ich Liebe Dich
11- Greek	Saghapo (inf), Ssaghapo (frm)
12- Hebrew	Ani Ohev Otach (to female)
	Ani Ohevet Otcha (to male)
13- Hindi	Mai tumse Pyar karta hoon (to female)
	Mai tumse Pyar karti hoon (to male)
14- Indonesian	Saya mencintaimu
15- Irish	Graimthu
16- Italian	Ti Amo
17- Japanese	Kimi O Ai Shiteru
18- Korean	Sarang hac
19- Portuguese	Eu Te Amo
20- Russian	ja teb'a l'ubl'u
21- Spanish	Te Amo, Te Quiero
22- Swahili	Ninaku Penda
23- Swedish	Jag A'Lskar Dig
24- Zulu	Ngiyakuthanda!

FILL IN THE ACTIVITY THAT YOU WANT <u>YOUR SPOUSE TO DO</u>

(Use your best handwriting.)
Make plenty of copies in different types of papers and colors.

Request For Pleasure & Excitement

Request: _____

_____

Date: _____ *Time*: _____

Place: _____

FILL IN THE ACTIVITY THAT <u>YOU WANT TO</u> DO FOR YOUR SPOUSE

This Voucher Is Good For One Event

I will.... _____

_____

Date: _____ *Time*: _____

FILL IN THE ACTIVITY THAT YOU WANT <u>YOUR SPOUSE TO DO</u>

(Use your best handwriting.)
Make plenty of copies in different types of papers and colors.

REQUEST FOR PLEASURE & EXCITEMENT

REQUEST: _____

_____

Date: _____ *Time*: _____

Place: _____

FILL IN THE ACTIVITY THAT <u>YOU WANT TO</u> DO FOR YOUR SPOUSE

THIS VOUCHER IS GOOD FOR ONE EVENT

I WILL... _____

_____

Date: _____ *Time*: _____

FILL IN THE ACTIVITY THAT YOU WANT <u>YOUR SPOUSE TO DO</u>

(Use your best handwriting.)
Make plenty of copies in different types of papers and colors.

Request For Pleasure & Excitement

Request: _____

_____

Date: _____ *Time*: _____

Place: _____

FILL IN THE ACTIVITY THAT <u>YOU WANT TO</u> DO FOR YOUR SPOUSE

This Voucher Is Good For One Event

I will... _____

_____

Date: _____ *Time*: _____

FILL IN THE ACTIVITY THAT YOU WANT <u>YOUR SPOUSE TO DO</u>

(Use your best handwriting.)
Make plenty of copies in different types of papers and colors.

Request For Pleasure & Excitement

Request: _____

_____

Date: _____ *Time:* _____

Place: _____

FILL IN THE ACTIVITY THAT <u>YOU WANT TO</u> DO FOR YOUR SPOUSE

This Voucher Is Good For One Event

I will... _____

_____

Date: _____ *Time:* _____

As A Man Thinks In His Heart, So Is He

Proverbs 23:7

Our life is what our thoughts make it.

– Marcus Aurelius

A man will find that as he alters his thoughts toward things, and other people, things and other people will alter towards him.

– James Allen

We are the sum total of what our thoughts are!!!

Wishing you good thoughts & a Life Filled With "Romance."

Benilda Nya

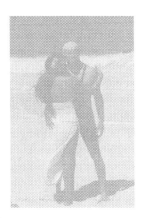

(Place one of your favorite pictures here of the two of you.)